D1154499

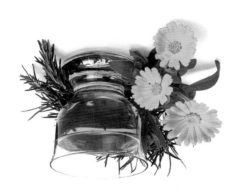

POCKET
MEDICINAL HERBS

PENELOPE ODY

A DK Publishing Book

Editor	Nasim Mawji
US Editor	Mary Sutherland
Designer	Robert Ford
Senior Art Editor	Tracey Clarke
DTP Designer	Harvey de Roemer
Managing Editor	Susannah Marriott
Managing Art Editor	Toni Kay
Production Controller	Patricia Harrington

First American Edition, 1997 2 4 6 8 10 9 7 5 3 1
Published in the United States by DK Publishing, Inc
95 Madison Avenue New York, New York 10016
Visit us on the World Wide Web at http://www.dk.com

Copyright © 1997 Dorling Kindersley Limited, London
Text copyright © 1997 Penelope Ody

All rights reserved under International and Pan-American Copyright
Conventions. No part of this publication may be reproduced, stored in a retrieval
system, or transmitted in any form or by any means, electronic, mechanical,
photocopying, recording, or otherwise, without the prior written permission of
the copyright owner. Published in Great Britain by Dorling Kindersley Limited.

Ody, Penelope
   Pocket Medicinal Herbs / by Penelope Ody. -- 1st American ed.
   p.   cm.
   Includes index.
   ISBN 0-7894-1616-6
   1. Herbs--Therapeutic use--Handbooks, manuals, etc. I. Title
RM666.H330386 1996
615'.321--dc20   96-30991
                          CIP

Reproduced by Flying Colours S.r.l in Italy
Printed and bound in Italy by LEGO

CONTENTS

INTRODUCTION

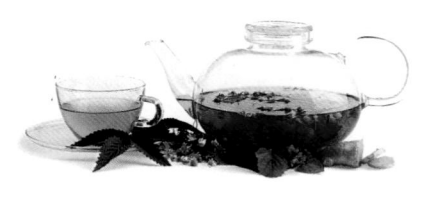

For centuries herbs were the primary means of
ensuring the family's health: favorite recipes were
handed down between generations, and local
healers were always ready to brew complex
concoctions for more troublesome ills. In many parts
of the world this is still the pattern of health care,
but for most Western civilizations the widespread
use of healing herbs in the home is a thing of the
past – or at least it was until quite recently.

❖

In the past decade there has been a
major resurgence of interest in making and using
herbal remedies – a growing popularity that can be
seen in the vast numbers of over-the-counter
herbal products now available from local
drugstores and supermarkets. Herbal remedies are
no longer the preserve of the herb supplier or
health food store; they have now
found a much wider audience.

Popularity can, however, breed confusion. Newcomers to herbs are faced with a bewildering array of exotic remedies that generally – because of stringent labeling laws – reveal very little of their actions or efficacy on the package. For those who prefer to grow their own herbs, the assortment of plants and seeds available from garden centers and nurseries can be equally confusing.

✧

Although many hundreds of healing herbs are used worldwide, most practicing herbalists limit their personal repertoire to about 100 plants. Indeed, some traditional healers argue that it is difficult to get to know and really understand more than half a dozen different herbs a year. Newcomers should thus take their herbal studies very slowly, while the more experienced should think very carefully before expanding their private *materia medica* to accommodate the latest fashionable fads.

✧

As a practicing herbalist I have often been asked by patients and herbal enthusiasts what my "top ten" herbs would be, or which dozen I might select for a medicinal herb garden. In this book I have tried to do just that: to choose a very limited selection of extremely versatile plants that can be combined to treat most minor ailments, and to select a core group for the amateur herbalist to focus on and start to understand.

✧

At the same time, this book also provides a portable guide to some of the most widely used herbs. Although the dozen *Key Medicinal Herbs* form the basis of most of the remedies, top-selling favorites that are found on the supermarket shelves – herbs such as echinacea, garlic, and devil's claw – are also covered.

✧

Worldwide, herbs still account for the majority of mankind's medicine; a surprisingly small number of plants could also do the same for many of us.

Penelope Ody

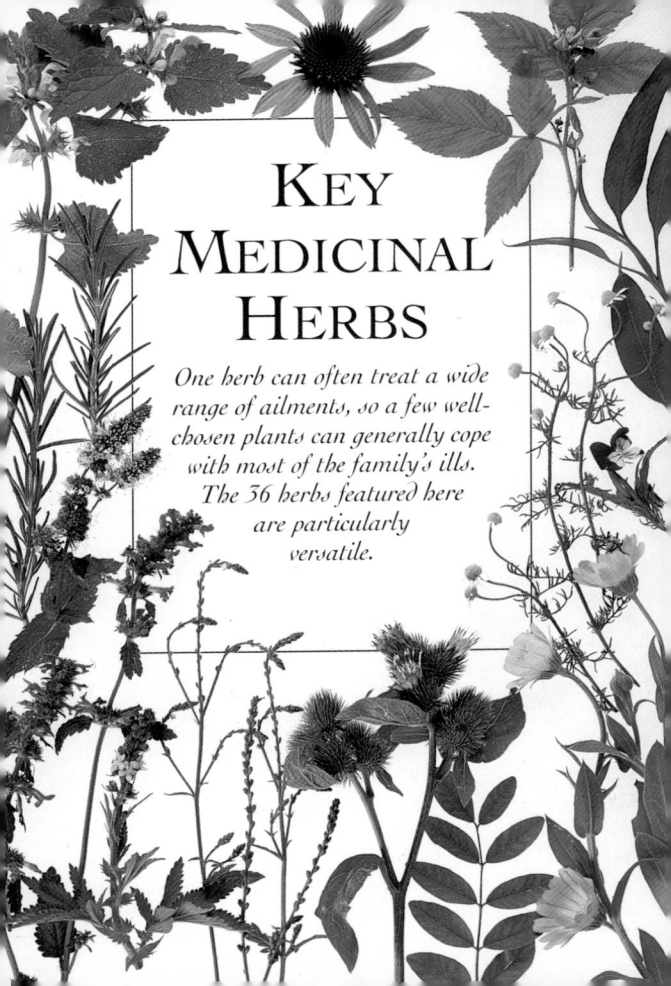

KEY
MEDICINAL
HERBS

One herb can often treat a wide
range of ailments, so a few well-
chosen plants can generally cope
with most of the family's ills.
The 36 herbs featured here
are particularly
versatile.

Achillea millefolium

YARROW

The Greek hero Achilles is believed to have used yarrow to cure battle injuries in the Trojan War – hence its botanical name and its ancient use as a wound herb.

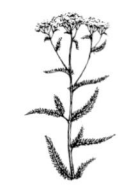

A perennial growing up to 12in (30cm).

KEY ACTIONS

- promotes sweating
- urinary antiseptic
- blood vessel relaxant
- anti-inflammatory
- stops bleeding

HOME REMEDIES

Infusion: Take for colds and flu (p. 64), and combine with other antiseptic herbs in cystitis remedies (p. 80). Use for poor circulation in the elderly (p. 83). Use externally in skin treatments (p. 79); also in compresses for varicose veins.

Fresh leaves: Insert into the nostril to stop a nosebleed.

Poultice: This can staunch bleeding wounds (p. 49).

OVER-THE-COUNTER

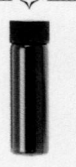

Essential oil: This deep-blue oil is antiallergenic, anti-inflammatory, and helpful in massage rubs for inflamed joints (p. 54). It can be used in steam inhalations for hay fever.

Tincture: Use as the infusion for colds and flu (p. 64), or take ½ tsp (2.5ml) 3 times a day with water.

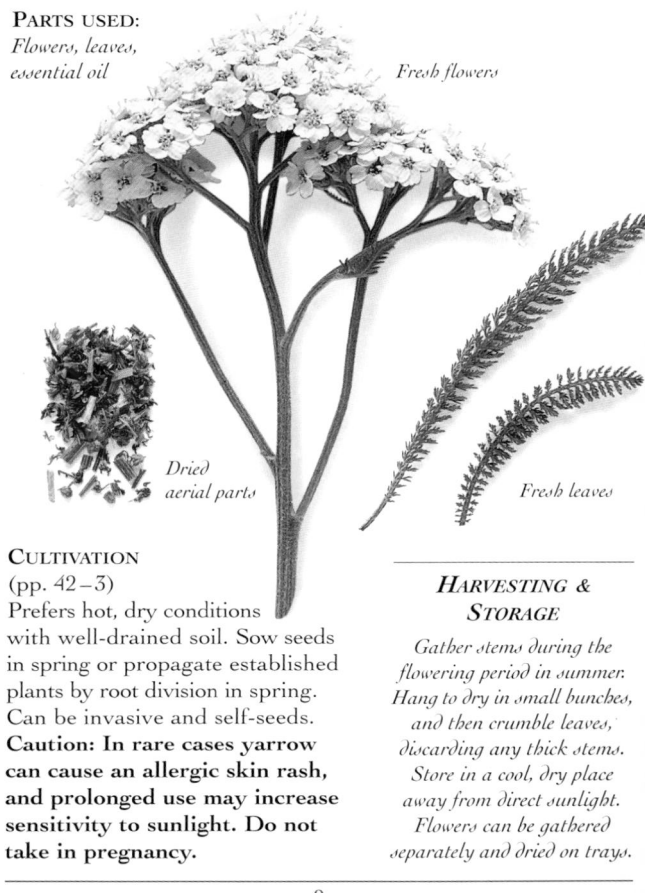

PARTS USED:
*Flowers, leaves,
essential oil*

Fresh flowers

*Dried
aerial parts*

Fresh leaves

CULTIVATION
(pp. 42–3)
Prefers hot, dry conditions
with well-drained soil. Sow seeds
in spring or propagate established
plants by root division in spring.
Can be invasive and self-seeds.
**Caution: In rare cases yarrow
can cause an allergic skin rash,
and prolonged use may increase
sensitivity to sunlight. Do not
take in pregnancy.**

HARVESTING &
STORAGE

*Gather stems during the
flowering period in summer.
Hang to dry in small bunches,
and then crumble leaves,
discarding any thick stems.
Store in a cool, dry place
away from direct sunlight.
Flowers can be gathered
separately and dried on trays.*

AGRIMONY

Agrimonia eupatoria

Mainly used today as a digestive remedy and astringent, agrimony was once more highly valued as a wound herb and was regularly used to treat battlefield injuries.

A perennial growing up to 24in (60cm).

KEY ACTIONS

- digestive & bile stimulant
- astringent
- diuretic
- heals wounds

HOME REMEDIES

🍵 *Infusion:* Take for indigestion (p. 68), diarrhea (p. 71) – especially in children – and food allergies. It is helpful for cystitis (p. 80) and heavy menstrual bleeding. It can also be used as a gargle for sore throats and nasal congestion, or to bathe sores, wounds, weeping eczema, and varicose ulcers.

📎 *Poultice:* Apply to relieve migraines and piles (p. 49).

OVER-THE-COUNTER

Tincture: More astringent and drying than an infusion, this is helpful for excess mucus or congestion. Take up to 4ml with water 3 times a day.

Tablets: Agrimony is found in digestive remedies and in treatments for piles. The herb is highly astringent so is best avoided if there is accompanying constipation.

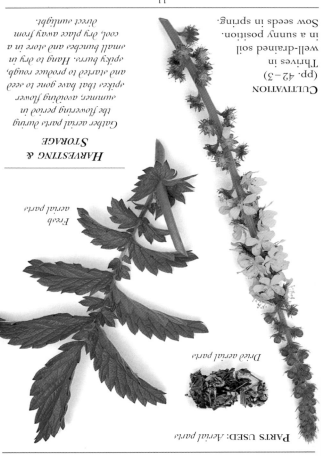

Sow seeds in spring.

CULTIVATION
(pp. 42–3)
Thrives in
well-drained soil
in a sunny position.

HARVESTING & STORAGE

Gather aerial parts during the flowering period in summer avoiding flower spikes that have gone to seed and started to produce rough, spiky burrs. Hang to dry in small bunches and store in a cool, dry place away from direct sunlight.

Fresh aerial parts

Dried aerial parts

PARTS USED: *Aerial parts*

AGRIMONY

Althaea officinalis

MARSH MALLOW

Marsh mallow has been regarded as a healing herb since ancient Egyptian times. The roots and leaves are extremely mucilaginous, or gluey, and help restore tissues.

A perennial growing up to 4ft (1.2m).

KEY ACTIONS

- soothing
- diuretic
- expectorant
- heals wounds

HOME REMEDIES

🫖 **Infusion**: Take for sinusitis, nasal congestion (p. 63), and cystitis (p. 80). For coughs, try the remedy on p. 66 or combine 500ml marsh mallow infusion with 500g honey to make a syrup (p. 67).

🐚 **Root powder**: Taken as a paste or in capsules with slippery elm powder, it eases digestive tract inflammation.

🍃 **Poultice**: This can help to draw out splinters (p. 49).

MACERATION
❖

The roots of herbs such as marsh mallow and valerian are more effectively macerated to extract active substances than decocted. Put 25g of dried root in a saucepan or bowl and add 500ml of cold water. Leave in a cool place overnight, then strain through a sieve or jelly bag. Marsh mallow root macerate soothes coughs and stomach inflammations – use with slippery elm powder instead of water (p. 69).

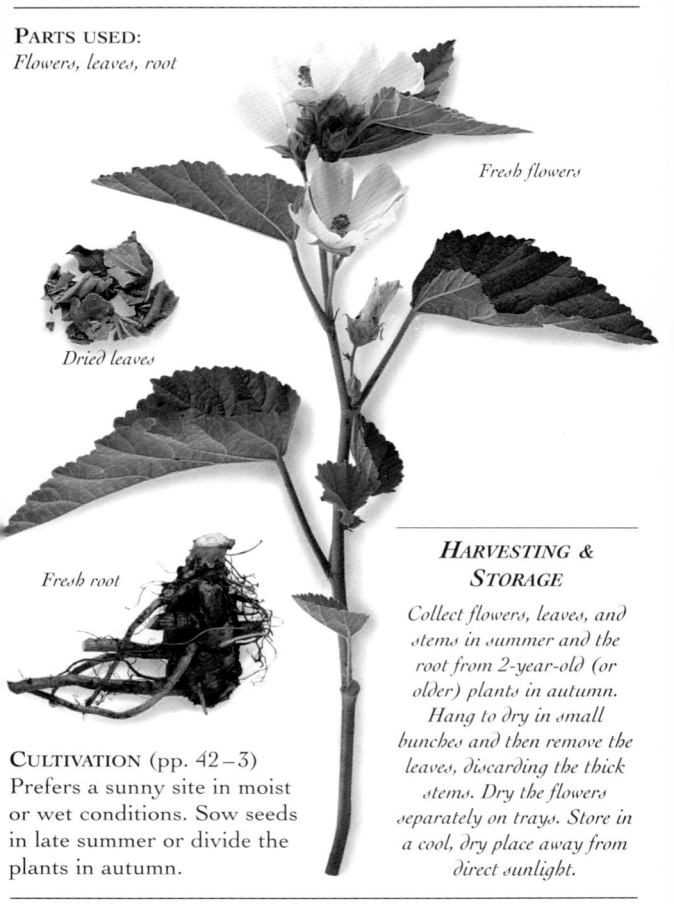

PARTS USED:
Flowers, leaves, root

Fresh flowers

Dried leaves

Fresh root

HARVESTING & STORAGE

Collect flowers, leaves, and stems in summer and the root from 2-year-old (or older) plants in autumn. Hang to dry in small bunches and then remove the leaves, discarding the thick stems. Dry the flowers separately on trays. Store in a cool, dry place away from direct sunlight.

CULTIVATION (pp. 42–3) Prefers a sunny site in moist or wet conditions. Sow seeds in late summer or divide the plants in autumn.

Calendula officinalis

Pot Marigold

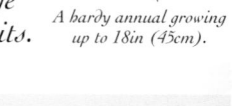

An effective antiseptic, pot marigold was used in medieval times to counter "plague and pestilence." Simply looking at its bright orange flowers was believed to lift the spirits.

A hardy annual growing up to 18in (45cm).

KEY ACTIONS

- astringent
- anti-inflammatory
- antimicrobial
- heals wounds

HOME REMEDIES

Infusion: Can be taken as a digestive stimulant and menstrual regulator. Use as a gargle for gum and throat infections or mouth ulcers (p. 73). Apply infusions externally in an eyebath for conjunctivitis and sties (p. 74) or for skin disorders (p. 79).

Infused oil: Soothes dry skin, eczema, piles, and fungal disorders such as yeast infections and athlete's foot.

OVER-THE-COUNTER
❖

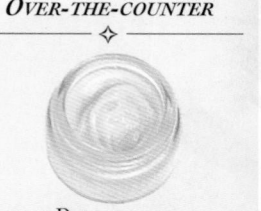

Cream: Patent creams and ointments are widely available (often under the Latin name *Calendula*). Use for minor skin injuries or inflammation, and eczema.

Tincture: Use as an alternative to infusions. Patent marigold tinctures may be made with 90% alcohol; avoid in pregnancy.

14

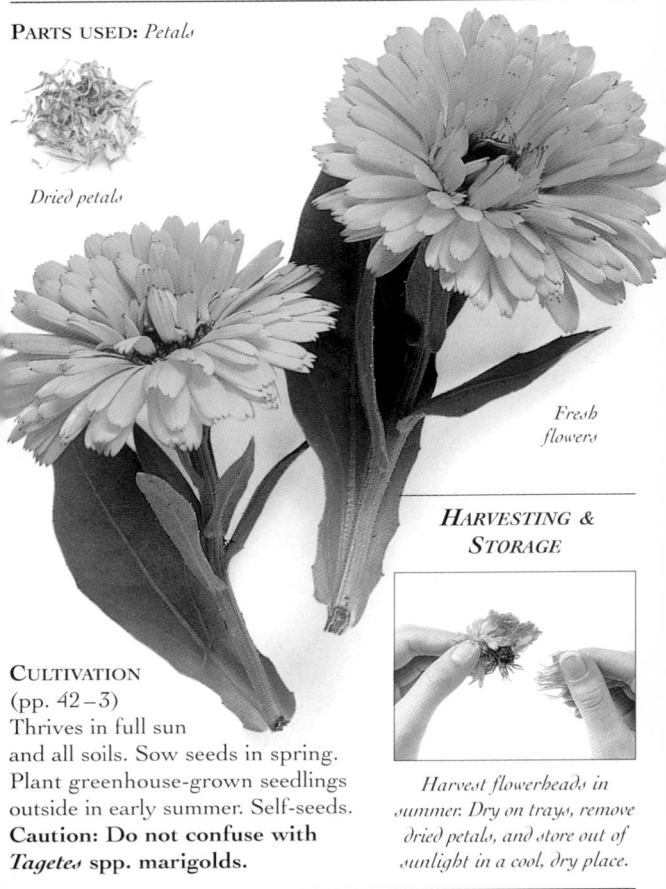

PARTS USED: *Petals*

Dried petals

Fresh flowers

HARVESTING & STORAGE

Harvest flowerheads in summer. Dry on trays, remove dried petals, and store out of sunlight in a cool, dry place.

CULTIVATION
(pp. 42–3)
Thrives in full sun and all soils. Sow seeds in spring. Plant greenhouse-grown seedlings outside in early summer. Self-seeds.
Caution: Do not confuse with *Tagetes* **spp. marigolds.**

Filipendula ulmaria

MEADOWSWEET

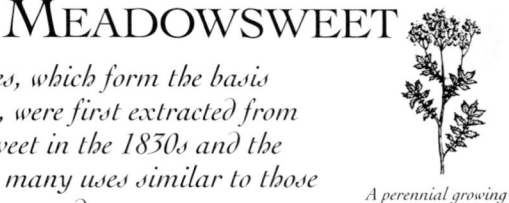

Salicylates, which form the basis of aspirin, were first extracted from meadowsweet in the 1830s and the plant has many uses similar to those of this common drug.

A perennial growing up to 4ft (1.25m).

KEY ACTIONS

- antirheumatic & anti-inflammatory
- promotes sweating
- calms digestion & soothes the stomach; antacid
- diuretic, mild urinary analgesic

HOME REMEDIES

Infusion: Take to relieve rheumatic pains (p. 59) and to ease feverish chills. Use for gastritis, stomach upsets, and irritable bowel problems (pp. 70, 89), and to counter food intolerance (p. 78). Applied as an eyewash, it relieves conjunctivitis and eye inflammation.

OVER-THE-COUNTER

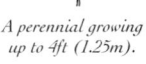

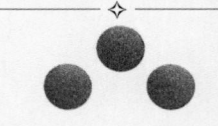

Tablets: Meadowsweet is used in many patent products, often combined with marshmallow to soothe gastritis, or with digestive stimulants such as dandelion.

Tincture: Convenient for travel first-aid kits: use to treat stomach upsets (p. 92). Take up to 1 tsp (5ml) 3 times a day with water.

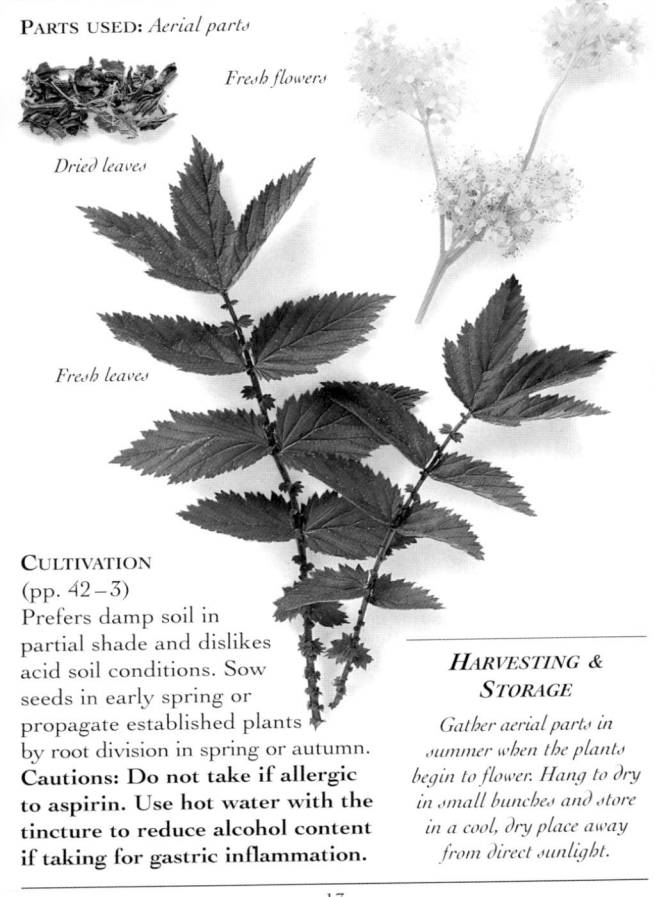

PARTS USED: *Aerial parts*

Fresh flowers

Dried leaves

Fresh leaves

CULTIVATION
(pp. 42–3)
Prefers damp soil in partial shade and dislikes acid soil conditions. Sow seeds in early spring or propagate established plants by root division in spring or autumn.
Cautions: Do not take if allergic to aspirin. Use hot water with the tincture to reduce alcohol content if taking for gastric inflammation.

HARVESTING & STORAGE

Gather aerial parts in summer when the plants begin to flower. Hang to dry in small bunches and store in a cool, dry place away from direct sunlight.

Hypericum perforatum

ST. JOHN'S WORT

Traditionally regarded as a wound herb, St. John's wort is now recognized as a potent antidepressant. It is widely prescribed by German doctors as an alternative to orthodox drugs.

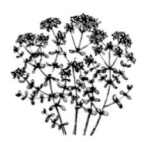

An upright plant growing up to 24in (60cm).

KEY ACTIONS

- mild analgesic
- antidepressant & sedative
- anti-inflammatory
- antiviral & astringent

HOME REMEDIES

Infusion: Take for menstrual pain (p. 81), menopausal symptoms (p. 82), anxiety, and depression. Drink or use in compresses to ease neuralgia (p. 76).

Infused oil: An essential standby for minor burns, cuts, and scrapes. Make with the flowering tops (p. 51) and use in rubs for muscular aches (p. 58) and in eardrops to soothe earache (p. 75).

MAKING OINTMENT

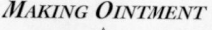

A simple ointment can be made easily by thickening the infused oil with beeswax. Melt 30g of beeswax in a double boiler or glass bowl over a pan of water. Warm 100ml of infused oil gently in a second double boiler, then add the warm oil to the beeswax. Stir well and pour into sterilized glass jars while still hot. Apply to minor burns, sunburn, cuts and scrapes, and inflamed joints.

PARTS USED: *Aerial parts, flowering tops*

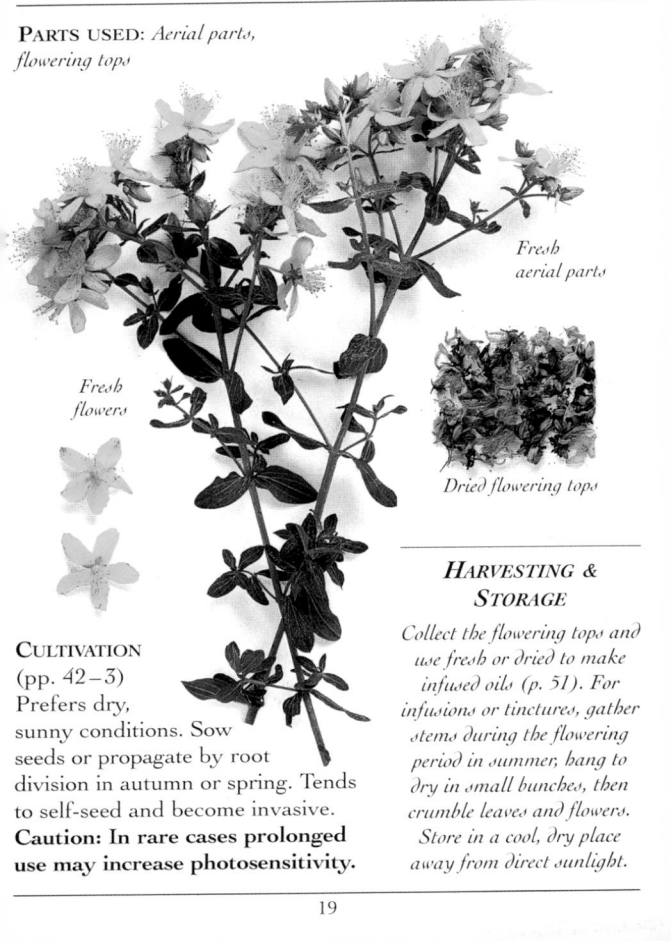

Fresh aerial parts

Fresh flowers

Dried flowering tops

CULTIVATION
(pp. 42–3)
Prefers dry, sunny conditions. Sow seeds or propagate by root division in autumn or spring. Tends to self-seed and become invasive.
Caution: In rare cases prolonged use may increase photosensitity.

HARVESTING & STORAGE

Collect the flowering tops and use fresh or dried to make infused oils (p. 51). For infusions or tinctures, gather stems during the flowering period in summer, hang to dry in small bunches, then crumble leaves and flowers. Store in a cool, dry place away from direct sunlight.

Lavandula angustifolia

LAVENDER

Used by the Romans to scent bath water, lavender's name derives from the Latin lavare, *to wash. It is one of the most popular medicinal herbs, valued as a cooling, calming remedy.*

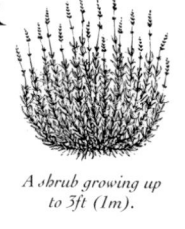

A shrub growing up to 3ft (1m).

KEY ACTIONS

- antispasmodic & carminative
- antibacterial & antiseptic
- antidepressant & nerve tonic
- topical circulatory stimulant

HOME REMEDIES

Infusion: Ideal for tension headaches (p. 77) and menopausal problems as well as insomnia, rheumatism, and digestive disorders. For a relaxing bath, add 1pt (500ml) to the bath water. A compress soaked in a hot infusion can help to relieve aching joints or earache (p. 75).

Infused oil: Cold infused oil (p. 51) is a useful substitute for the essential oil.

OVER-THE-COUNTER
⋄

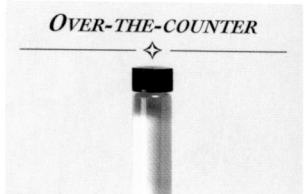

Essential oil: Massage into the temples for migraines (p. 77) or use in a steam inhalation for congestion (p. 63) and laryngitis or in facial steamers (p. 79). Apply pure oil to cold sores or add to rubs for coughs (p. 66), muscular aches (p. 58), or to bring relief during labor (p. 85).

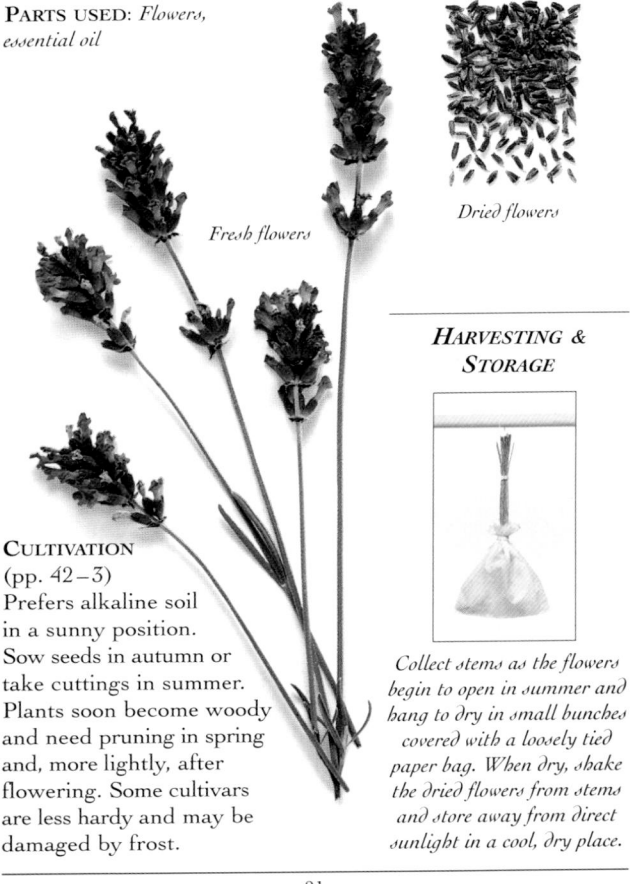

PARTS USED: *Flowers, essential oil*

Fresh flowers

Dried flowers

CULTIVATION
(pp. 42–3)
Prefers alkaline soil
in a sunny position.
Sow seeds in autumn or
take cuttings in summer.
Plants soon become woody
and need pruning in spring
and, more lightly, after
flowering. Some cultivars
are less hardy and may be
damaged by frost.

HARVESTING & STORAGE

*Collect stems as the flowers
begin to open in summer and
hang to dry in small bunches
covered with a loosely tied
paper bag. When dry, shake
the dried flowers from stems
and store away from direct
sunlight in a cool, dry place.*

Matricaria recutita & Chamaemelum nobile

CHAMOMILE

*German chamomile (M. recutita)
and Roman chamomile (C. nobile)
are both used medicinally. The herb
was once known as "ground apple"
because of its distinctive smell.*

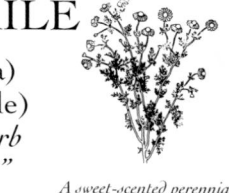

*A sweet-scented perennial
growing to 18in (45cm).*

KEY ACTIONS

- bitter & prevents vomiting
- antibacterial & antiseptic
- anti-inflammatory
- carminative
- sedative

HOME REMEDIES

Infusion: Drink as a
soothing remedy for nausea
and digestive disorders (p. 68)
or as a calming bedtime drink.
Add to a toddler's bath water
to encourage sleep (p. 86).

Dried flowers: Steam
releases anti-inflammatory and
antiallergenic chemicals
present in the flowers. Use in
inhalations to counter hay fever
or mild asthma attacks (p. 66).

OVER-THE-COUNTER

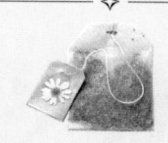

Teabags: Used teabags
can soothe tired eyes
(p. 75) and ease earache.
Essential oil: This can be
expensive, but 1–2 drops
will suffice for most uses.
Add to bath water to ease
tension (p. 61) or use
instead of dried flowers in
steam inhalations. It can
also soothe teething babies
(p. 87). Avoid in pregnancy.

PARTS USED: *Flowers*

Fresh flowers

Dried flowers

CULTIVATION
(pp. 42–3)
Prefers well-drained,
slightly acidic, moist
or dry soil in full sun.
Sow seeds in spring or
autumn. Both single- and
double-flowered varieties
can be used medicinally.

**HARVESTING &
STORAGE**

*Collect the flowers when
they first open and use
fresh or dry on trays. Store
in a cool dry place. The
flowers soon deteriorate with
drying, and freezing can be
better for long-term storage.*

Rosmarinus officinalis

ROSEMARY

Herbalists have long regarded rosemary as a potent tonic and believed it could "gladden the harte." It is warming and has a stimulating effect on the nervous system.

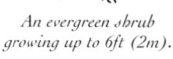

An evergreen shrub growing up to 6ft (2m).

KEY ACTIONS

- tonic & stimulant nervine
- circulatory & heart tonic
- antibacterial & antiseptic
- antidepressant
- carminative

HOME REMEDIES

Infusion: A stimulating tonic drink said to improve concentration and memory (p. 61). Use as a hair rinse for dandruff and scalp psoriasis (p. 79) or as a color enhancer for dark hair. Rinse or gargle with it to ease mouth, gum, or throat infections (p. 73).

Infused oil: Hot infused oil (p. 50) can be substituted for essential oil in massage rubs.

OVER-THE-COUNTER

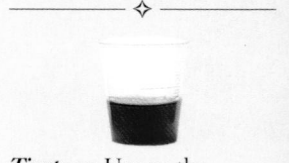

Tincture: Use as the infusion. Take up to ½ tsp (2.5ml) 3 times daily or gargle with 1 tsp (5ml) diluted in a glass of water 3–4 times a day.

Essential oil: Use in rubs for arthritis and muscular aches (p. 58); in a warm compress for headaches. Diluted oil can soothe teething babies (p. 87).

PARTS USED: *Flowers, leaves, essential oil*

Fresh aerial parts

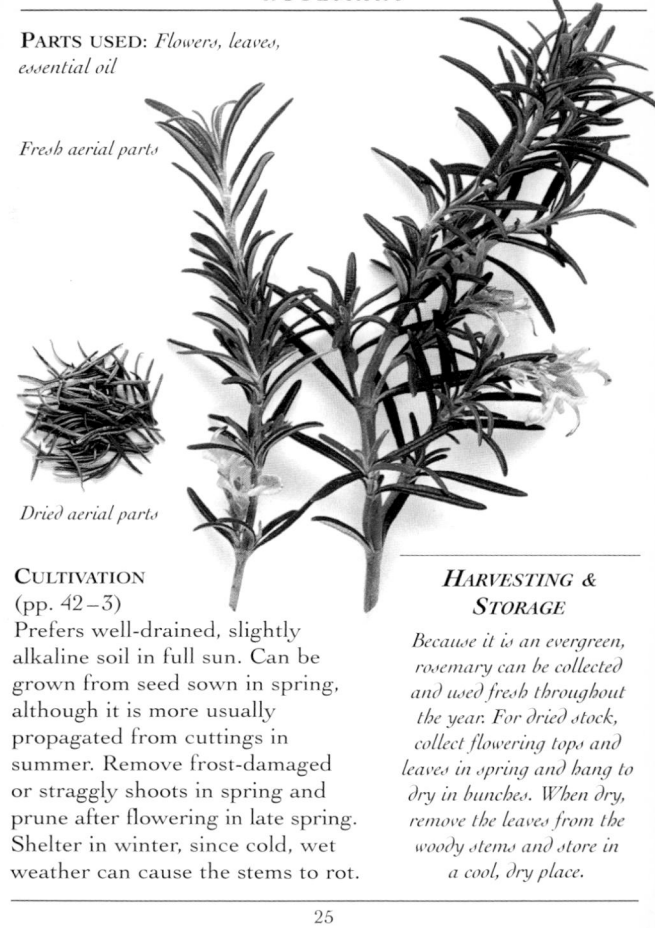

Dried aerial parts

CULTIVATION
(pp. 42–3)
Prefers well-drained, slightly alkaline soil in full sun. Can be grown from seed sown in spring, although it is more usually propagated from cuttings in summer. Remove frost-damaged or straggly shoots in spring and prune after flowering in late spring. Shelter in winter, since cold, wet weather can cause the stems to rot.

HARVESTING & STORAGE

Because it is an evergreen, rosemary can be collected and used fresh throughout the year. For dried stock, collect flowering tops and leaves in spring and hang to dry in bunches. When dry, remove the leaves from the woody stems and store in a cool, dry place.

25

Stachys officinalis

WOOD BETONY

Once a favorite Anglo-Saxon healing herb, wood betony has fallen from use in recent years, but it is an attractive plant, useful for treating liver and nervous disorders.

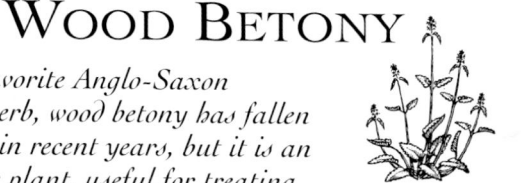

A perennial growing up to 2ft (60cm).

KEY ACTIONS

- mild sedative & tonic
- cerebral circulation tonic
- bitter digestive remedy
- astringent

HOME REMEDIES

Infusion: One of the more palatable herb teas; take for headaches (p. 77) or nervous tension and insomnia (p. 60). Long associated with women's health, it helps to ease labor pains and period cramps. It also stimulates circulation to the brain in the elderly. Take as a liver tonic or for food intolerance (p. 78) and use externally to bathe infected wounds and sores.

MAKING TINCTURES

◆

Place 100g dried herb in a large screw-top jar and cover with 335ml vodka (37.5% proof) and 165ml water (this produces a 25% alcohol/water mixture). Shake the mixture every couple of days for 2 weeks, then strain the mixture (usually brown) through a jelly bag or wine press. Store in a clean glass bottle for up to 2 years. Typical dosage is 5ml 3 times a day. Use as the infusion.

PARTS USED: *Aerial parts*

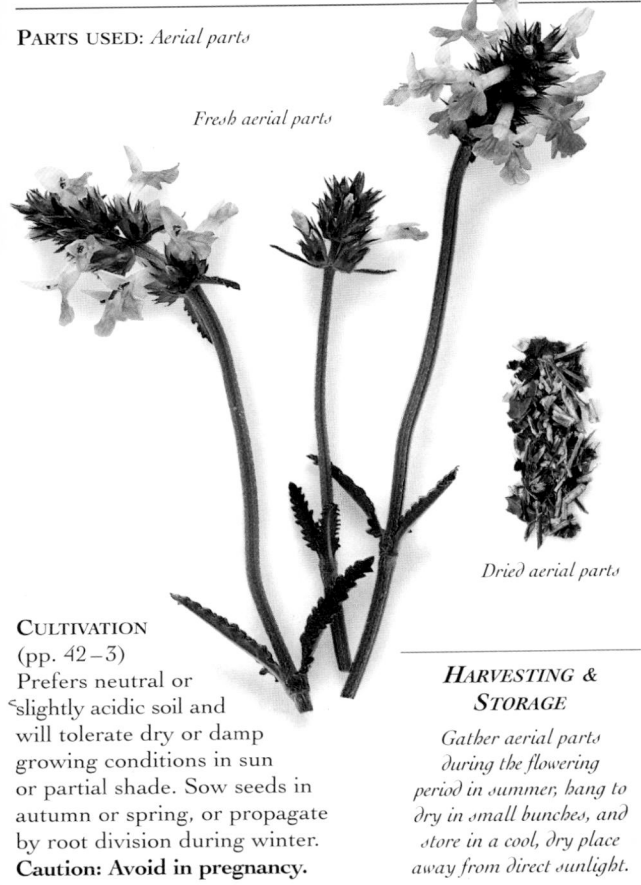

Fresh aerial parts

Dried aerial parts

CULTIVATION
(pp. 42–3)
Prefers neutral or
slightly acidic soil and
will tolerate dry or damp
growing conditions in sun
or partial shade. Sow seeds in
autumn or spring, or propagate
by root division during winter.
Caution: Avoid in pregnancy.

HARVESTING & STORAGE

*Gather aerial parts
during the flowering
period in summer, hang to
dry in small bunches, and
store in a cool, dry place
away from direct sunlight.*

Thymus vulgaris

THYME

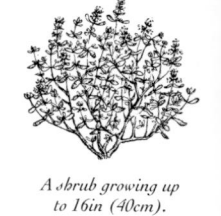

A potent antiseptic, thyme has long been used to treat lung infections. The name may derive from a Greek word for courage, indicating its use as a stimulating tonic.

A shrub growing up to 16in (40cm).

KEY ACTIONS

- antiseptic, antimicrobial & antiviral
- antispasmodic & carminative
- stimulating tonic
- expectorant

HOME REMEDIES

Infusion: Useful as a gargle for mouth and throat infections. It can also be taken for chest infections, diarrhea, and irritable bowel syndrome, and as a tonic for fatigue.

Syrup: Take for dry irritable coughs, whooping cough, or bronchitis (p. 67).

Infused oil: Use the hot infused oil (p. 50) as an alternative to the essential oil.

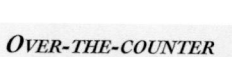

OVER-THE-COUNTER

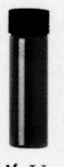

Essential oil: Useful as an antiseptic for treating infections. Use in chest rubs for coughs and congestion (p. 66) or for muscular aches (p. 58). Diluted oil can soothe insect stings and infected wounds. A few drops in a hot bath can ease rheumatic pains.

PARTS USED: *Aerial parts, essential oil*

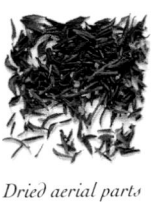

Dried aerial parts

CULTIVATION
(pp. 42–3)
Intolerant of wet
soil in winter.
Propagate from
seed sown in spring,
from cuttings taken in
summer, or by dividing
established plants in late
summer. Has a tendency
to become woody after a
couple of years, so prune
hard in early spring and
clip lightly after flowering
to encourage new growth.
**Caution: Avoid high doses
in pregnancy.**

*Fresh aerial
parts*

HARVESTING & STORAGE

*Collect aerial parts during
flowering in summer and
hang to dry in small
bunches. When dry, crumble
leaves and smaller stems and
store in clean glass jars in a
cool, dark, dry place. Harvest
fresh sprigs throughout the
growing season.*

Verbena officinalis

VERVAIN

Regarded as sacred by both the Romans and Druids, vervain was once believed to have magical properties. Today it is mainly used for nervous disorders and liver problems.

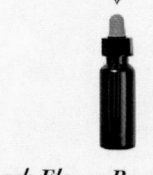

A perennial growing up to 2ft 6in (80cm).

KEY ACTIONS

- bile stimulant
- relaxing & sedative
- uterine stimulant
- promotes sweating & milk flow

HOME REMEDIES

Infusion: Use as a liver restorative in many conditions, including hay fever (p. 62). It is helpful for anxiety, nervous tension (p. 60), and emotional problems associated with menopause (p. 82).

Fresh leaves: Crushed leaves soothe insect stings.

Poultice: Apply a poultice for sprains and strains (p. 49).

Ointment: Useful for neuralgia, wounds, and sores.

OVER-THE-COUNTER

Bach Flower Remedy: Vervain is recommended for mental stress and over-exertion, insomnia, and an inability to relax.

Teabags: Improve liver function and digestion, while encouraging rest and sleep.

Tincture: Use as the infusion. Take up to 1 tsp (5ml) 3 times a day.

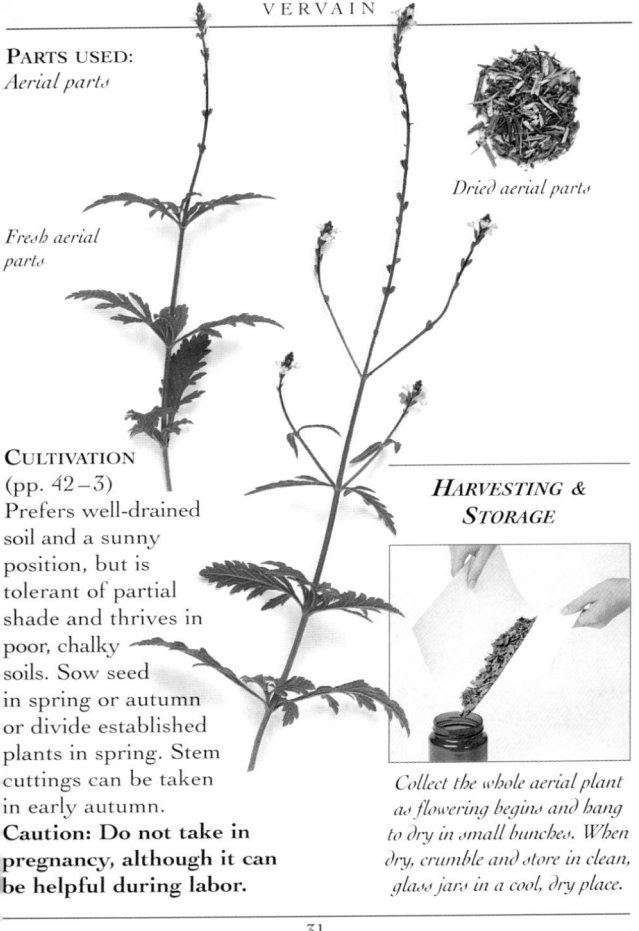

PARTS USED:
Aerial parts

Dried aerial parts

Fresh aerial parts

CULTIVATION
(pp. 42–3)
Prefers well-drained soil and a sunny position, but is tolerant of partial shade and thrives in poor, chalky soils. Sow seed in spring or autumn or divide established plants in spring. Stem cuttings can be taken in early autumn.
Caution: Do not take in pregnancy, although it can be helpful during labor.

HARVESTING & STORAGE

Collect the whole aerial plant as flowering begins and hang to dry in small bunches. When dry, crumble and store in clean, glass jars in a cool, dry place.

TONIC HERBS

Used for thousands of years to boost energy levels and once regarded as sacred, many tonic herbs are now widely available in over-the-counter remedies.

DANG GUI

CHINESE ANGELICA,
DONG QUAI, TANG KWAI
*Angelica polymorpha
var. sinensis*

Part used: Root

Key actions:
Analgesic, blood
tonic, antispasmodic,
circulatory stimulant,
laxative, uterine stimulant.

Key uses: Used to treat anemia
and menstrual problems; a
good women's tonic,
especially after childbirth.

Caution: Avoid in pregnancy.

GOTU KOLA

INDIAN PENNYWORT
Centella asiatica

Parts used:
Aerial parts

Key actions:
Bitter, blood tonic

and purifier, digestive tonic,
diuretic, relaxant, laxative.

Key uses: Long used as a
rejuvenating remedy to
counter problems of old age
and improve failing memory.
Makes a stimulating tea for
times of stress or fatigue.

SIBERIAN GINSENG

Eleutherococcus senticosus

Part used: Root

Key actions:
Antistress,
antiviral,
reduces
blood sugar,
adrenal
stimulant,
circulatory
stimulant, aphrodisiac,
immune stimulant.

Key uses: Can provide extra
energy and can help the body

to cope in the approach to a stressful period. It can help jet lag (p. 93) as well as chronic fatigue syndrome. Also used to help counter the toxic effects of chemotherapy and radiation treatment. A gentler alternative to Korean ginseng, it may be a preferred choice for women.

REISHI
LING ZHI,
RED LACQUERED
BRACKET FUNGUS
Ganoderma lucidem

Parts used: Fruiting body of the fungus
Key actions: Antibacterial, antitumor, antiviral, expectorant, reduces high blood pressure, immune stimulant, sedative.
Key uses: A Taoist energy tonic for long life, also used to treat liver disorders. It can lower blood sugar and cholesterol levels and can be an effective tonic for the over-anxious or elderly.

KOREAN GINSENG
REN SHEN, KING PLANT
Panax ginseng

Part used: Root
Key actions: Immune stimulant, tonic, reduces blood sugar and cholesterol levels, aphrodisiac, heart tonic.
Key uses: Rich in steroidal compounds similar to human sex hormones, hence its use as an aphrodisiac. A useful winter energy tonic, it can also aid recovery from chest problems.
Caution: Avoid caffeine.

DAMIANA
CURZON
Turnera diffusa
var. *aphrodisiaca*

Parts used: Aerial parts
Key actions: Aphrodisiac, diuretic, antidepressant, reviving, mood enhancer.
Key uses: A stimulant and a useful tonic in convalescence, it is also helpful for menstrual and prostate problems.

KITCHEN REMEDIES

The kitchen cupboard can provide a wealth of herbal remedies for treating minor ailments or for emergency first aid if more orthodox treatments are unavailable.

ONION
Allium cepa

Key actions: Antibiotic, cleansing, expectorant, reduces blood sugar and cholesterol levels.

Key uses: Hot onions and pepper can be given for colds to encourage sweating and reduce fevers. Apply raw to insect stings and warts.

CABBAGE
Brassica oleracea

Key actions: Anti-inflammatory, antibacterial, liver restorative.

Key uses: Used for a range of problems, including acne, arthritis, digestive problems, chest infections, migraines, water retention, and mastitis (p. 85). Bandage a crushed leaf to aching arthritic joints. In Germany it is used in some cancer therapies.

TEA
Camellia sinensis

Key actions: Astringent, antioxidant, antibacterial.

Key uses: Black tea can help counter diarrhea and dysentery; green tea is known to help reduce tooth decay and strengthen the immune system. Apply used green tea teabags directly to cuts and scrapes to stop bleeding or to soothe insect stings. Oolong tea is reputed to reduce cholesterol and improve digestion.

CINNAMON
Cinnamon zeylanicum

Key actions: Digestive and circulatory stimulant.

Key uses: Sold powdered or in sticks, made from the inner bark, cinnamon is a warming remedy for colds and chills (p. 64), indigestion, colic, and diarrhea. The Chinese believe that cinnamon bark strengthens kidney energy and the twigs improve peripheral circulation.

LEMON
Citrus limon

Key actions: Detoxifying, antibacterial.

Key uses: Boosts the immune system, counters infection, and can relieve rheumatic pains and neuralgia (apply externally). Dilute fresh juice with water as a gargle for sore throats.

FENNEL
Foeniculum vulgare

Key actions: Digestive tonic, carminative, expectorant, anti-inflammatory.

Key uses: Eases indigestion, colic, and stomach upsets. The seeds stimulate milk flow in nursing mothers, so drinking fennel infusion while breast-feeding can both improve milk flow/supply and provide a weak colic remedy (p. 87).

NUTMEG
Myristica fragrans

Key actions: Carminative, antispasmodic.

Key uses: Grated nutmeg soothes digestive upsets and chronic diarrhea. Use the oil in massage rubs for rheumatic aches and pains, muscle strain, or during labor (p. 85). Substitute for sage oil to relieve toothache (p. 87).

Caution: In high doses (over 7.5g) it is hallucinogenic and may cause convulsions.

OTHER USEFUL HERBS

*The 12 key medicinal herbs (pp. 8–31) and the 24 in this chart
provide a practical and versatile selection of herbs for home use.*

Parts used listed in **bold** after common and botanical names; glossary p. 96.

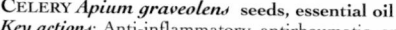

GARLIC *Allium sativum* **cloves, oil**
Key actions: Antimicrobial, bile stimulant, expectorant, immune stimulant, reduces blood cholesterol and blood sugar levels.
Key uses: Internally – heart and circulatory tonic, mucus, infections, digestive disorders. Externally – acne, corns, warts, verrucas, fungal infections (fresh cloves). **Cautions**: Avoid high doses during breast-feeding and pregnancy; can irritate sensitive stomachs. Avoid heavily deodorized products.

CELERY *Apium graveolens* **seeds, essential oil**
Key actions: Anti-inflammatory, antirheumatic, antispasmodic, carminative, diuretic, increases uric acid excretion, urinary antiseptic.
Key uses: Internally – rheumatism, arthritis, and gout; cystitis and urinary disorders; high blood pressure; increases milk flow in nursing mothers. Externally – arthritis (oil). **Cautions**: Avoid in pregnancy; the essential oil can increase skin photosensitivity; do not take seeds for cultivation internally.

BURDOCK *Arctium lappa* **leaves, seeds, root**
Key actions: Cleansing, laxative, diuretic, promotes sweating, antirheumatic, antibacterial (seeds), reduces blood sugar level (seeds).
Key uses: Internally – rheumatic and skin disorders (root, leaves); colds and feverish chills (seeds). Externally – skin sores and inflammation (poultices); varicose ulcers (infused oil). **Notes**: Included in patent remedies for acne and minor skin problems, often with dandelion or nettles.

ECHINACEA *Echinacea angustifolia, E. pallida, E. purpurea* **aerial parts, root**
Key actions: Antiallergenic, antimicrobial, anti-inflammatory, immune stimulant, lymphatic tonic, raises white blood cell count, heals wounds.
Key uses: Internally – colds, flu, sore throats; kidney infections; food poisoning; glandular fever; acne, boils. Externally – skin infections, wounds, infected insect bites (creams and ointments). **Caution**: High doses can cause nausea and dizziness.

EUCALYPTUS *Eucalyptus globulus* leaves, essential oil

Key actions: Antimicrobial, antispasmodic, antiviral, expectorant, febrifuge, expels worms, reduces blood sugar level. *Key uses*: Externally – bronchitis, coughs, lung infections, joint and muscular pain (massage oils); nasal and bronchial congestion (inhalations); sore throats, wounds (infusion as a wash). *Notes*: Dilute essential oil for massage rubs or add 10 drops to gargles and steam inhalations; powdered leaves are sold in capsules.

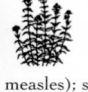

BONESET *Eupatorium perfoliatum* aerial parts

Key actions: Antispasmodic, bitter, promotes sweating, febrifuge, immune stimulant, laxative. *Key uses*: Internally – feverish chills, common cold, flu, childhood fevers (including chicken pox and measles); severe bone pains; liver stagnation, sluggish digestion. *Notes*: Often included in patent decongestant and hay fever remedies. *Caution*: High doses may cause vomiting.

LICORICE *Glycyrrhiza glabra* root, juice

Key actions: Adrenal tonic, antiallergenic, anti-inflammatory, antiviral, expectorant, laxative, reduces blood cholesterol level, soothes gastric mucosa, tonic. *Key uses*: Internally – arthritis; gastric inflammation and ulcers; asthma, bronchitis, and chest coughs. Aids recovery after steroid treatment. *Cautions*: Avoid excessive or prolonged use with high blood pressure, pregnancy, liver cirrhosis, or if taking digoxin-based drugs.

HOPS *Humulus lupulus* strobules from the female plant

Key actions: Anaphrodisiac, antiseptic, antispasmodic, astringent, bitter, diuretic, mild analgesic, nerve tonic, sedative. *Key uses*: Internally – nervous tension, anxiety, insomnia; irritable bowel syndrome; premature ejaculation; loss of appetite; menopausal emotional upsets. Externally – ulcers and slow-healing wounds (infusion as a wash). *Cautions*: Avoid with depression; growing plants may cause contact dermatitis.

HYSSOP *Hyssopus officinalis* aerial parts, essential oil

Key actions: Decongestant, antispasmodic, antiviral, carminative, diuretic, expectorant, promotes sweating, sedative. *Key uses*: Internally – colds, flu, sore throats; digestive upsets; nervous stomachs; bronchitis; coughs; anxiety. Externally – eczema and bruises (infusion as a wash); bronchitis, coughs, nervous exhaustion, melancholy (oil in rubs and baths). *Caution*: Excessive use of essential oil can cause convulsions.

ELECAMPANE *Inula helenium* **flowers, root**
Key actions: Decongestant, antiseptic, antispasmodic, digestive stimulant, expectorant, promotes sweating, tonic. *Key uses*: Internally – bronchitis, asthma, hay fever, stubborn coughs, flu, respiratory problems; digestive tonic and liver stimulant. Externally – skin rashes, varicose ulcers (infusion as a wash). *Notes*: An effective tonic after flu or in long-standing respiratory disorders; often included in commercial cough syrups.

WILD LETTUCE *Lactuca virosa* **leaves, dried juice (latex)**
Key actions: Anaphrodisiac, mild analgesic, antispasmodic, mild hypnotic, relaxing nervine, sedative. *Key uses*: Internally – nervous excitability, anxiety, insomnia, hyperactivity in children; persistent irritant or nervous coughs. *Notes*: Often combined with hops and passion flower in insomnia products. Latex was once sold as a substitute for opium. *Caution*: Excess may cause restlessness.

WHITE DEADNETTLE *Lamium album* **flowering tops**
Key actions: Anti-inflammatory, decongestant, antispasmodic, astringent, diuretic, expectorant, menstrual regulator, styptic, heals wounds. *Key uses*: Internally – cystitis; heavy or irregular periods; prostate problems; irritable bowel syndrome. Externally – piles, minor cuts and scrapes (infusion as wash); conjunctivitis (infusion as eyebath). *Notes*: Tea can help recovery after surgery for benign prostate enlargement.

LEMON BALM *Melissa officinalis* **aerial parts, essential oil**
Key actions: Antibacterial, antispasmodic, antidepressant, antiviral, carminative, digestive stimulant. *Key uses*: Internally – indigestion; melancholy; nervous exhaustion, stress; fevers, chills. Externally – swellings (compress); insect bites, insect repellent (cream). *Notes*: The essential oil is used in massage oils for depression, anxiety, and chest congestion; included in products for anxiety and insomnia, often with valerian.

PEPPERMINT *Mentha* x *piperita* **aerial parts, essential oil**
Key actions: Antispasmodic, carminative, digestive tonic, mild sedative, prevents vomiting, relaxes peripheral blood vessels, promotes sweating. *Key uses*: Internally – indigestion, poor appetite, digestive upsets, gall bladder problems, colitis, nausea, vomiting. Externally – Excess mucus, bronchial congestion (oil); skin irritations, fungal infections (infusion as wash). *Cautions*: May irritate mucous membranes; not to be given to babies or when breast-feeding.

PLANTAIN & ISPHAGHULA *Plantago lanceolata, P. major, P. ovata* leaves (ribwort and common plantain), seeds (isphaghula)

Key actions: Ribwort – decongestant, expectorant; common – antibacterial, blood tonic, diuretic, stops bleeding, expectorant; isphaghula – demulcent, laxative. *Key uses*: Ribwort – congestion, inflamed mucous membranes; common – diarrhea, irritable bowel syndrome, insect bites, sore throats; isphaghula – constipation, irritable bowel syndrome.

RASPBERRY *Rubus idaeus* leaves, fruit

Key actions: Antispasmodic, astringent, preparative for childbirth, digestive stimulant, tonic. *Key uses*: Internally – to ease childbirth, menstrual pain, and heavy menstrual bleeding; mild diarrhea. Externally – sores, wounds, varicose ulcers (infusion as wash); sore throats, gum disease (leaf infusion as mouthwash/gargle); sore eyes (infusion as eyebath). *Caution*: Avoid high doses of leaves until the last 2 months of pregnancy.

YELLOW DOCK *Rumex crispus* root

Key actions: Bile stimulant, bitter, cleansing tonic, laxative. *Key uses*: Internally – liver congestion and related digestive problems; irritant skin eruptions, boils; rheumatic disorders. Externally – mouth ulcers (infusion as mouthwash). *Notes*: Included in many remedies for skin rashes, including eczema and boils; also in laxative mixtures.

SAGE *Salvia officinalis* leaves, essential oil

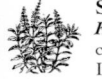

Key actions: Antiseptic, antispasmodic, astringent, bile stimulant, carminative, reduces perspiration, salivation and milk flow. *Key uses*: Internally – tonic; menopausal night sweats; improves digestion and circulation; reduces milk flow at weaning. Externally – sore throats, mouth ulcers, gum disorders (infusion as gargle/mouthwash); insect bites, sores (ointment). *Cautions*: High doses should be avoided by epileptics and in pregnancy.

ELDER *Sambucus nigra* flowers, leaves, berries, bark

Key actions: Diuretic, laxative, promotes sweating; decongestant, expectorant, circulatory stimulant, topical anti-inflammatory (flowers). *Key uses*: Internally – feverish colds, flu, excess mucus; prophylactic for hay fever, sore throats, mouth ulcers (flowers). Externally – chapped skin, sores, chilblains, eye inflammations (flowers); wounds (leaves). *Caution*: The bark is a purgative and should be avoided in pregnancy.

SKULLCAP *Scutellaria lateriflora* aerial parts

Key actions: Antibacterial, antispasmodic, cooling, digestive stimulant, lowers cholesterol levels, relaxing nervine, sedative. *Key uses*: Internally – for anxiety; nervous exhaustion, stress, and excitability; premenstrual tension; migraine; insomnia; helpful in programs for withdrawal from addictive tranquilizers. *Notes*: Widely used in sedative and insomnia mixtures, often combined with hops and valerian.

DANDELION *Taraxacum officinale* leaves, root, sap

Key actions: Antiseptic, bitter digestive tonic, diuretic, reduces blood cholesterol levels, urinary antiseptic; laxative and bile stimulant (root). *Key uses*: Internally – skin and rheumatic disorders; liver congestion and digestive weakness; indigestion; poor appetite. Externally – warts (fresh sap). *Notes*: Added to heart remedies as a source of potassium and to improve blood flow to the liver; often sold in patent products for fluid retention.

VALERIAN *Valeriana officinalis* root

Key actions: Allays pain, antispasmodic, carminative, reduces blood pressure, tranquilizer. *Key uses*: Internally – anxiety; insomnia; palpitations; high blood pressure; migraine, tension headaches; menstrual pain; bronchial spasm. Externally – muscle cramps (compress); sores, wounds, and ulcers (infusion as wash). *Cautions*: Prolonged use can cause headaches and palpitations; avoid with other sleep-inducing drugs.

HEARTSEASE *Viola tricolor* aerial parts

Key actions: Anti-inflammatory, antirheumatic, diuretic, expectorant, laxative, stabilizes capillary membranes. *Key uses*: Internally – eczema; acne; helps prevent capillary hemorrhage; bronchitis, whooping cough. Externally – cradle cap in babies, weeping sores, insect bites, and skin rashes (cream or ointment, infusion as wash). *Note*: Rich in saponins so high doses can cause nausea and vomiting.

GINGER *Zingiber officinalis* root, essential oil

Key actions: Prevents vomiting, antispasmodic, antiseptic, carminative, circulatory stimulant, anti-inflammatory, expectorant, promotes sweating. *Key uses*: Internally – nausea, morning sickness; poor appetite; colic, indigestion, irritable bowel syndrome; colds; flu; poor circulation; menstrual cramps. Externally – rheumatic pains (hot infused oil). *Notes*: Tablets and capsules sold for motion sickness; ginger beer or candy also effective.

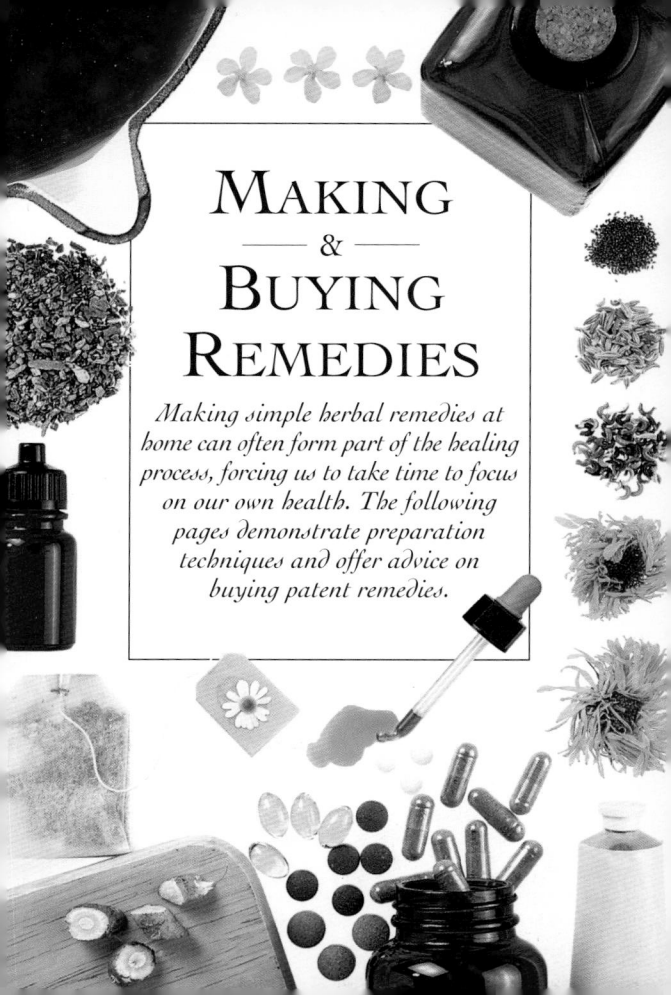

MAKING
— & —
BUYING
REMEDIES

Making simple herbal remedies at home can often form part of the healing process, forcing us to take time to focus on our own health. The following pages demonstrate preparation techniques and offer advice on buying patent remedies.

GROWING HERBS

Many herbs are easy to grow and will often flourish in poor soil if the site is sunny. Many of the key herbs (pp. 8–31) grow well in temperate climates.

BUYING PLANTS

Some herbs are slow-growing so consider buying established plants from a herb nursery.

• Buy plants in late spring when the danger of frost is past and nurseries still have stocks of young, healthy plants.
• Look for strong, healthy specimens with plenty of new growth and space in the pot.

• Avoid straggling, yellowing herbs in weed-choked pots or with roots emerging from the base. Loose soil suggests recent replanting.
• Examine the underside of leaves for pests such as aphids, red spider mite, and whitefly.
• Try to check that plants are correctly labeled – mistakes can and do happen.

GROWING PLANTS

Growing herbs in a window box or garden is easy and satisfying.

FROM SEED
It is best to sow annual and biennial herbs directly where they are intended to grow, following packet instructions. Celery, chamomile, dill, and pot marigold are easy to grow. Perennials that grow well from seed include elecampane, fennel, feverfew, hyssop, sage, wood betony, catnip, thyme, St. John's wort, ribwort plantain, and skullcap. White deadnettle, dandelion, and chickweed grow as weeds.

BY ROOT DIVISION

Divide roots with a small fork or sharp spade in early spring. Replant immediately and water thoroughly. Roman chamomile, peppermint, and elecampane can be propagated by cutting and replanting the small offsets and runners.

FROM CUTTINGS

Woody perennial herbs are best propagated by cuttings taken from side shoots in late summer or early autumn. Dip the base of the shoot in hormone rooting powder and pot. Try elder, hyssop, thyme, lavender, rosemary, and sage.

WHEN TO HARVEST

Choose a dry day and gather herbs once the morning dew has gone. The leaves of evergreens, such as hyssop and rosemary, can be collected anytime except on frosty days.

EARLY SPRING	**Roots**: dandelion.
LATE SPRING	**Flowers**: elder.
EARLY TO MIDSUMMER	**Flowers/flowering tops**: chamomile, pot marigold, St. John's wort. **Aerial parts/leaves before flowering**: agrimony, catnip, dandelion, dill, feverfew, hyssop, lemon balm, peppermint, plantain, raspberry, sage.
MID-TO LATE SUMMER	**Aerial parts while flowering**: boneset, chickweed, comfrey, heartsease, marsh mallow, meadowsweet, passion flower, peppermint, skullcap, thyme, vervain, white deadnettle, wild lettuce, wood betony, yarrow. **Flowers**: hops, lavender. **Leaves**: ginkgo.
AUTUMN	**Roots/bulbs when the leaves have wilted**: burdock (first year), echinacea, elecampane (2–3-year-old roots), garlic, marsh mallow, valerian, yellow dock, fennel. **Seeds or fruit when ripe**: celery, chaste tree, dill, elder, evening primrose.

DRYING HERBS

Seasonal growing patterns inevitably limit the availability of fresh herbs and mean that they need to be gathered, dried, and stored for future use.

Dry herbs quickly to avoid losing the valuable aromatic constituents through evaporation, and to limit deterioration due to oxidation. Herbs should be dried away from direct sunlight in a place where plenty of air can circulate. A ventilated cupboard, a sunny room, or a dry garden shed with a low-powered fan are all suitable. Avoid using a garage as herbs can become contaminated with gasoline fumes. Keep the drying room between 70–90°F (20–32°C).

It is possible to dry herbs within 5 or 6 days; the longer it takes, the more likely the plant is to discolor and lose its flavor. Do not dry herbs in microwave ovens; this may alter their chemical make up.

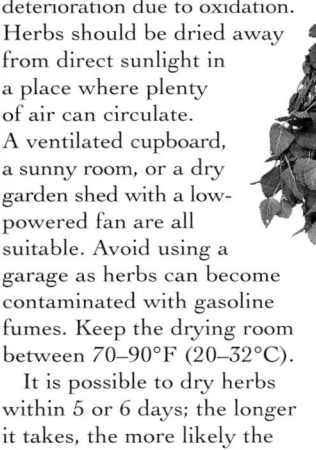

Leaves and aerial parts should be hung by the stems in small bunches. When dry, crumble the leaves, including smaller pieces of stem if required.
Stems bearing smaller flowers or seeds, such as dill or lavender, can be hung in small bunches. Cover with a paper bag to catch falling seeds.

Large flowers, such as pot marigolds, are best cut from stems and dried on trays in a ventilated cupboard.

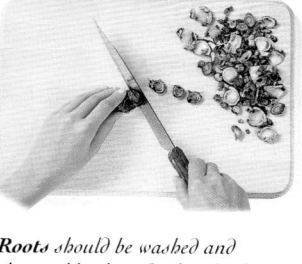

Roots should be washed and thoroughly cleaned when fresh, then chopped into small pieces and dried on trays in a cupboard or cooling oven.

Bulbs, such as garlic, need to be dug up in the autumn once aerial parts have died down.

Bark should be collected in autumn, taking care not to remove too much from any section of the tree or bush. Collect small pieces, wipe clean, then chop and dry as for roots.

Berries should be collected when ripe and dried as for roots.

BUYING DRIED HERBS

Not all herbs can be grown in every climate, and garden space can be limited, so buying dried herbs is often necessary.

• Choose a reputable store or specialty mail-order supplier.
• Always buy the minimum quantity you need and store in dark glass or pottery jars.
• Look for bright colors and strong smells. Herbs tend to lose their color and aroma with age and poor storage, and drab, dusty-looking herbs are usually well past their prime.
• Sunlight makes herbs deteriorate, so avoid those stored in clear glass jars.
• Try to check that the herbs supplied are correctly labeled, as mistakes do happen. Some herbs have obvious visual clues (characteristic seed pods in skullcap, for example); others have distinctive smells.
• Poorly harvested and stored herbs can easily become contaminated: check for mouse droppings, signs of mold, insect infestation, or excessive amounts of other plant material such as dried grass.

MAKING INFUSIONS

Herbal infusions are an easy way to take medicinal herbs. They can be drunk hot or cold and sweetened with a little honey, if desired.

1 *Warm a teapot or jug with hot water and add the fresh or dried herbs. Pour on freshly boiled water, put the lid on the teapot or jug, and allow to infuse for 10 minutes.*

PARTS USED: *fresh or dried leaves, flowers, most aerial parts of herbs, and small seeds.*

EQUIPMENT: *kettle; teapot or jug with a close-fitting lid; plastic or nylon tea strainer; tea cup.*

STANDARD QUANTITIES: *25g dried herbs or 75g fresh herbs to 500ml of water; no more than 30g herbs to 500ml water for a combination of dried herbs.*

STANDARD DOSAGE: *one cup or wineglass 3 times a day. Reheat before each dose or drink cold.*

STORAGE: *make enough for 1 day and store in a covered jug in a cool place.*

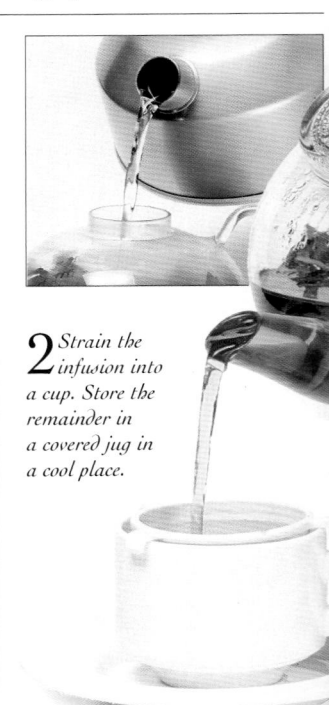

2 *Strain the infusion into a cup. Store the remainder in a covered jug in a cool place.*

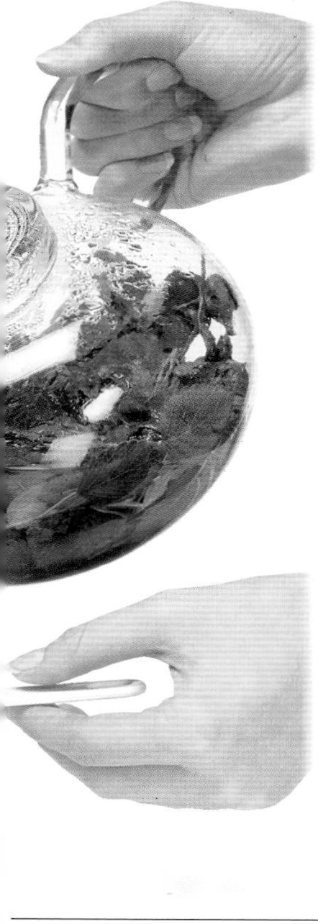

TISANE CUPS

To make a single-cup infusion:

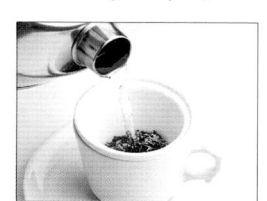

1 Put 2 tsp of dried herbs into the strainer, pour on freshly boiled water, and cover with the lid.

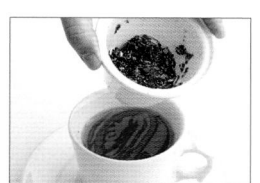

2 Allow to infuse for 10 minutes, then remove the strainer.

TEABAGS

Commercially produced herbal teabags are widely available or try tying 1–2 tsp of dried herbs in a small 4in square piece of muslin. Infuse in a cup of freshly boiled water for 10 minutes.

MAKING DECOCTIONS

The tougher parts of plants need to be decocted or simmered in water to extract their healing constituents; a gentler process is maceration (p. 12).

PARTS USED: *fresh or dried berries, seeds, bark, and roots.*

EQUIPMENT: *saucepan (stainless steel, enamel, glass, ceramic, or fireproof pottery, but not aluminum); plastic or nylon strainer; jug with a lid.*

STANDARD QUANTITIES: *25g dried herbs or 75g fresh herbs to 750ml of water, which reduces to 500ml after simmering. For a combination of herbs, the total weight should not exceed 30g herbs to 750ml water.*

STANDARD DOSAGE: *one cup or wineglass 3 times a day. Reheat before each dose or drink cold if preferred. A little honey or lemon juice can help improve the flavor.*

STORAGE: *make enough for 1 day and store in a covered jug in a cool place.*

1 *Put the herbs in a saucepan with the water and bring to a boil. Simmer for 20–40 minutes or until the volume has reduced by a third.*

COMBINED DECOCTION/INFUSION

This method is used to combine berries, bark, and roots with flowers or leaves in a mixture. See recipes for quantities.

Strain through a sieve

1 Put the berries, bark, or roots in a saucepan and cover with 750ml of cold water.

2 Simmer until the mixture has reduced by a third.

3 Place the dried flowers or leaves for the infusion in a teapot or lidded jug.

4 Strain the decoction onto the dried herbs in the teapot or jug and allow to infuse for 10–15 minutes.

5 Strain into a cup and sweeten with honey or unrefined sugar if desired.

2 Strain the mixture into a jug and store the surplus in a covered jug in a cool place.

MAKING A POULTICE

Fresh herbs, or plants such as cabbage, can be applied directly to minor injuries or ailments in a poultice. Chop the herb, boil it for 5 minutes, then squeeze out any surplus liquid.

Smooth oil on the affected area to prevent sticking, then spread the herb mixture on. Secure the poultice in position with gauze or cotton strips. Reapply every 2–4 hours.

MAKING INFUSED OILS

Infused oils are an easy-to-make alternative to creams and ointments, and form an ideal base for massage oils and chest rubs.

HOT INFUSED OILS

1 *Put the herbs and oil into the top half of a double saucepan or a glass bowl over a saucepan of water. Simmer for 3 hours, refilling the lower saucepan as required.*

PARTS USED: *dried leaves and aerial parts, roots.*

EQUIPMENT: *double saucepan or glass bowl and saucepan; muslin bag and wine press, or jelly bag; large jug; airtight, sterilized dark glass bottles; funnel (optional).*

STANDARD QUANTITIES: *200g dried herbs to 500ml sunflower oil.*

STORAGE: *store in sterilized dark glass bottles in a cool place and out of direct sunlight for up to a year.*

Muslin bag

Wine press

2 *Strain the hot infused mixture through a wine press or jelly bag into a jug. Store in dark glass bottles.*

COLD INFUSED OILS

1 *Tightly pack the jar with the herbs and cover with oil. Exposed herbs are liable to get moldy, so fill up with oil as required. Seal the jar and leave on a sunny windowsill for at least 2 weeks.*

Oil to cover

Jelly bag

PARTS USED: *dried flowers and petals.*

EQUIPMENT: *large glass screw-top jar; muslin bag and wine press, or jelly bag; large jug; airtight, sterilized dark glass storage bottles; funnel (optional).*

STANDARD QUANTITIES: *enough herb to fill the jar and sufficient cold-pressed sunflower, safflower, or walnut oil to cover.*

STORAGE: *as for hot infused oils.*

2 *Pour the mixture through a wine press or jelly bag to extract the oil. Store in dark glass bottles in a cool place.*

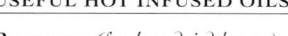

USEFUL HOT INFUSED OILS	USEFUL COLD INFUSED OILS

Rosemary *(fresh or dried leaves) for aches and pains.*
Comfrey *(dried leaves) for bruises, sprains, and arthritis.*
Chickweed *(dried aerial parts) for irritant eczema.*

St. John's wort *(fresh flowering tops) for sunburn, minor scalds and burns, scrapes, and inflamed joints.*
Pot marigold *(fresh or dried petals) for scratches, eczema, yeast infections, and athlete's foot.*

BUYING REMEDIES

The pressures of modern life may leave no time to brew tinctures or blend creams, but fortunately, a good selection of herbal products is available over the counter.

TABLETS & PILLS

Pills often use lactose (milk sugar) as a base and these should be avoided by anyone allergic to dairy produce. Pills may be coated in sugar to disguise the taste or have an enteric coating that is resistant to stomach acid, preventing them from dissolving until they reach the lower bowel. This is helpful with herbs like garlic that may cause stomach irritation. Typical dosage is generally the equivalent of 600mg of dried herb daily.

CAPSULES

Many companies package single herbs – typically echinacea, garlic, devil's claw, ginseng, and ginkgo – in capsules. These usually contain 200mg of herb powder, occasionally reinforced with concentrated extracts, giving the equivalent of up to 2g of herb. Herb combinations are also available. Check an herb's actions in a comprehensive herbal if in doubt or take professional advice. Dosage is typically up to 600mg 3 times a day. If capsules are difficult to swallow, separate the gelatin segments and take the powder with ½ tsp of honey or in a little water.

TINCTURES

These herbal extracts are made by soaking plant material in a mixture of alcohol and water and then pressing the brew to obtain a liquid, which is normally brown or dark green (to make, see p. 26). Tinctures are usually sold in dropper bottles and are often highly priced. Herbalists may use up to 20 herbs in a tincture mixture, although most prefer to limit the mix to no more than 5 herbs. Typical dosages range from 10–20 drops to 5–10ml, 3 times a day. Higher doses can often be beneficial: up to 10ml of echinacea 3 times a day is ideal for colds. Tinctures are usually taken before meals; they should be diluted in warm water and may be sweetened with a little honey.

TEABAGS

Commercial teabags can contain stale herbs of dubious quality, but many suppliers offer single sampling bags, which allow you to check quality and taste before buying in bulk.

Teabags usually contain small quantities of several herbs so, for therapeutic use, look for single herb teabags (fennel, peppermint, elderflower, and vervain are common) and use a combination of 2 or 3 for each cup. Store-bought teabags are often flavored with dried fruits, which are best avoided by those on low-sugar diets.

See page 45 for advice on buying dried herbs.

JUICES

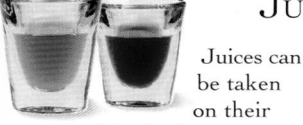

Juices can be taken on their own, combined with tinctures or used topically on the skin in lotions. Common commercially made juices include chamomile, dandelion, oat, echinacea, lemon balm, onion, rosemary, sage, St. John's wort, thyme, valerian, and yarrow. Dosage is usually 10ml 2–3 times a day, sweetened with honey if desired. Bottles of juice should be refrigerated once opened.

SYRUPS

Soothing for coughs and sore throats, syrups are a combination of herbal extracts and sugar, which acts as a preservative. Popular herbs for commercial cough syrups include licorice, thyme, hyssop,

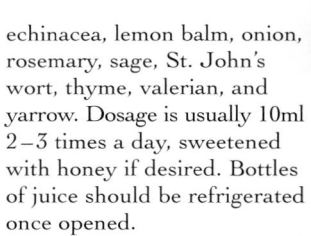

marsh mallow, and elecampane as well as less familiar herbs such as ipecac and squills, which are both potent expectorants. Dosage is typically 5–10ml of syrup 3–4 times a day.

ESSENTIAL OILS

Highly concentrated herb extracts, essential oils are commonly adulterated with synthetic substitutes, so be sure to buy from a reputable supplier.

Most essential oils can irritate the skin and should be diluted with either water, vegetable oils (such as sweet almond oil), wheat germ oil, and sunflower oil, or with an infused herbal oil (pp. 46–7). Use 5–6 drops of essential oil in a bath. For a massage oil, blend 1–2 drops with each 1ml of carrier oil.

CREAMS

Combining fats, oils, and water-based substances, creams are readily absorbed and soften the skin. Most commercial preparations use a complex mixture of organic fats and petroleum-derived bases, and may contain preservatives to improve shelf life.

OINTMENTS

Ointments contain fats and oils but no water, so they do not readily soak into or soften the skin but form a protective layer over it, encouraging healing. They are ideal when the sore area is likely to be regularly in contact with moisture, as in diaper rash. Patent ointments usually have petroleum jelly or paraffin wax as a base and contain natural fats and oils, including lanolin.

USEFUL CREAMS & OINTMENTS

Arnica for bruises, sprains, and chilblains (only if the skin is unbroken).

Chamomile for eczema and allergic skin conditions.

Chickweed for irritant eczema and to draw corns, boils, or splinters.

Comfrey for bruises, sprains, and arthritis (only if skin is unbroken).

Elderflower for chapped hands.

Evening primrose for dry skin and eczema.

Heartsease for diaper rash and skin rashes.

Pot marigold for cuts, scrapes, dry eczema, and fungal infections.

Sage for insect stings and as a general antiseptic first-aid cream.

Slippery elm as a drawing ointment for splinters and corns.

Tea tree as an antiseptic and for fungal infections.

Witch hazel in astringent creams for piles or varicose veins.

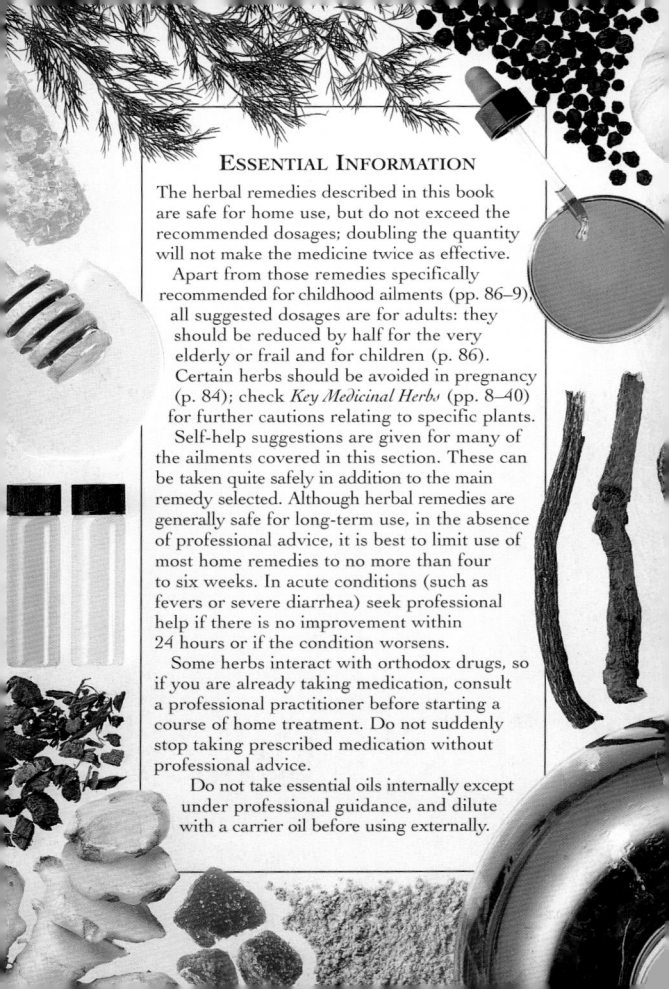

ESSENTIAL INFORMATION

The herbal remedies described in this book
are safe for home use, but do not exceed the
recommended dosages; doubling the quantity
will not make the medicine twice as effective.

Apart from those remedies specifically
recommended for childhood ailments (pp. 86–9),
all suggested dosages are for adults: they
should be reduced by half for the very
elderly or frail and for children (p. 86).
Certain herbs should be avoided in pregnancy
(p. 84); check *Key Medicinal Herbs* (pp. 8–40)
for further cautions relating to specific plants.

Self-help suggestions are given for many of
the ailments covered in this section. These can
be taken quite safely in addition to the main
remedy selected. Although herbal remedies are
generally safe for long-term use, in the absence
of professional advice, it is best to limit use of
most home remedies to no more than four
to six weeks. In acute conditions (such as
fevers or severe diarrhea) seek professional
help if there is no improvement within
24 hours or if the condition worsens.

Some herbs interact with orthodox drugs, so
if you are already taking medication, consult
a professional practitioner before starting a
course of home treatment. Do not suddenly
stop taking prescribed medication without
professional advice.

Do not take essential oils internally except
under professional guidance, and dilute
with a carrier oil before using externally.

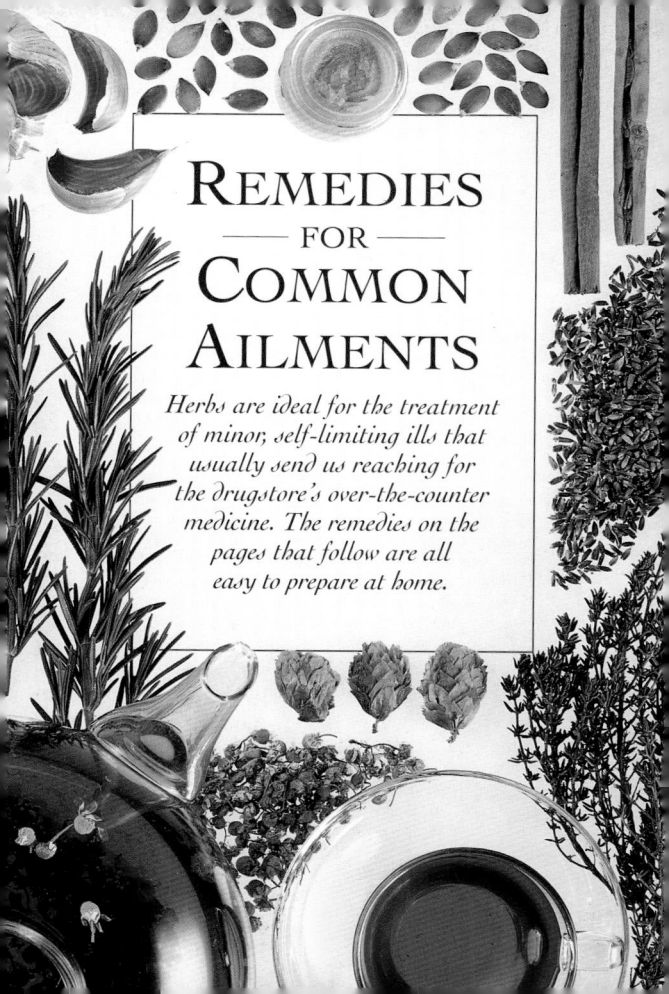

REMEDIES
— FOR —
COMMON
AILMENTS

Herbs are ideal for the treatment of minor, self-limiting ills that usually send us reaching for the drugstore's over-the-counter medicine. The remedies on the pages that follow are all easy to prepare at home.

ACHES & PAINS

Rather than acting as superficial painkillers to relieve symptoms, herbal remedies for aches and pains treat the causes — by improving circulation, ridding the body of irritant toxins, and repairing damaged tissues.

LAVENDER & ROSEMARY RUB

TO RELIEVE MUSCULAR ACHES & PAINS

Gentle massage with this simple combination of oils can ease stiffness and pain.

- 10 drops lavender oil
- 10 drops rosemary oil
- 10 drops thyme oil
- 19ml infused St. John's wort oil*

Method: Add the essential oils to the St. John's wort oil in a 20ml sterilized, dark glass bottle; shake well.

Application: Pour ½ tsp of the oil onto one palm, rub it between the palms, and gently massage the aching area. Repeat at least twice a day.

*See caution p. 19.

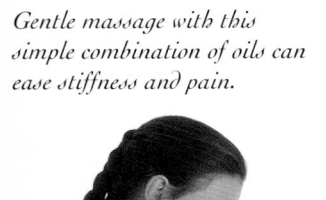

MEADOWSWEET & BURDOCK TEA

FOR ACHES & PAINS ASSOCIATED WITH ARTHRITIS

A cleansing mixture to help clear the toxins contributing to arthritis and ease stiffness in the joints.

- 60g dried meadowsweet*
- 20g each of yarrow* and celery seed,* both dried
- 50g each of dried burdock root, dried yellow dock* root and dried elderberries (mixed)

Method: Mix the meadowsweet, yarrow, and celery seed. Make a decoction (pp. 48–9) with 15g of the root and berry mixture and 750ml of water. Strain onto 10g of the herb mixture in a teapot; infuse for 10 minutes. **Dosage:** One cup 3 times a day before meals. Reheat before each dose.

*See cautions pp. 17, 9, 36, 39.

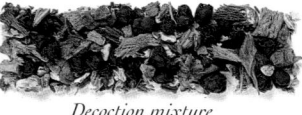

Decoction mixture   *Infusion mixture*

SELF-HELP SUGGESTIONS
❖

Massage comfrey cream or oil into arthritic joints to help repair old damage caused by previous injuries.

Avoid refined carbohydrates and animal products, which leave acid wastes in the body and can aggravate arthritis.

DEVIL'S CLAW

Kalahari bushmen used devil's claw for aches and pains. Research has identified it as a potent anti-inflammatory, analgesic, and antirheumatic agent. It has proved an effective remedy for arthritis. Take up to 600mg in capsules up to 3 times daily for at least 6 weeks. Avoid in pregnancy.

ANXIETY & FATIGUE

Occasionally, the tensions caused by stress and worries can be overwhelming; herbal sedatives can provide a gentle and nonaddictive alternative to powerful tranquilizing drugs.

SKULLCAP & WOOD BETONY TEA

To Relieve Tension & Treat Insomnia

Relaxing herbs can relieve tensions and form the basis of nighttime teas for insomnia.

- 40g dried skullcap
- 20g dried wood betony✿
- 20g dried vervain✿
- 10g dried lemon balm

Method: Mix the herbs and use 2 tsps per cup to make an infusion (pp. 46–7). For insomnia, replace the wood betony and lemon balm with 15g each of dried hops and dried St. John's wort✿ **Dosage:** Up to 4 cups daily as a remedy for anxiety, or 1 cup of the alternative mix 30 minutes before bedtime for insomnia. Sweeten this with honey since hops are bitter.

✿See cautions pp. 27, 31, 37, 19.

Vervain

Lemon balm

Skullcap

Wood betony

GOTU KOLA & DAMIANA TEA

STIMULATING TEA TO COMBAT FATIGUE

Tonic herbs in stimulating teas are a less aggressive option to caffeine-based brews.

- 15g dried gotu kola
- 10g damiana
- 5g fresh or dried rosemary

Method: Mix the herbs and make an infusion (pp. 46–7).

Dosage: One cup 3 times a day before meals.

Damiana

Gotu kola

Rosemary

SELF-HELP SUGGESTIONS

If a stressful period is looming, take up to 600mg of Siberian ginseng in capsules daily to improve the body's ability to cope.

Add up to 5 drops of lavender or chamomile essential oil to baths at night to encourage relaxation.

Deep breathing for 10 minutes a day can aid relaxation.

Take up to 500mg of valerian 3 times daily for anxiety, nervous tension, and insomnia.

Take up to 600mg of St. John's wort 3 times daily as an antidepressant. See caution p. 19.

PASSION FLOWER

The Aztecs used passion flower as a purgative; other Native Americans regarded the root as a blood tonic. The aerial parts are sedative and widely available in over-the-counter products for insomnia and stress. Take 200mg up to 3 times daily or a 400mg dose at night.

CONGESTION

Congestion often heralds a cold but may also be associated with sinus inflammation, or dust and pollen allergies. Herbal inhalations can bring relief and longer-term use of teas can ease chronic problems.

ELDERFLOWER & DANDELION TEA
FOR THE TREATMENT OF HAY FEVER

Herbs that strengthen the mucous membranes and cleanse the liver of toxins help the body to cope with allergies.

Dandelion

- 10g dandelion root
- 5g licorice root*
- 25g each of dried elderflowers, dried vervain,* and dried hyssop (mixed)

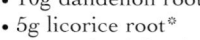
Vervain

Method: Make a decoction (pp. 48–9) with the roots and 750ml of water. Strain onto 15g of the herb mixture and infuse for 10 minutes.
Dosage: One cup 3 times a day before meals for 3–4 weeks during early spring.
*See cautions pp. 37, 31.

Hyssop

LAVENDER & THYME INHALATION

FOR CLEARING MUCUS & SOOTHING SINUSITIS

Steam inhalations using astringent and antiseptic herbs can help combat congestion.

- 4ml lavender oil
- 3ml thyme oil
- 2ml tea tree oil
- 20 drops peppermint oil*

SELF-HELP SUGGESTIONS

◇

Relieve sore and itching eyes associated with hay fever with a well-strained marigold infusion (pp. 46–7) used in an eye bath.

To relieve congestion at night, add a few drops of lavender, peppermint, or thyme essential oil to a saucer of water by the bed, or use in a diffuser.

For nasal congestion, massage elderflower cream into the sinus areas morning and night.

For sinusitis, drink an infusion (pp. 46–7) of ribwort plantain and marsh mallow leaves 3 times daily.

Method: Mix the essential oils in a 10ml sterilized, dark glass dropper bottle and shake well.

Application: Add 10 drops of the mixture to a basin of boiling hot water. Lean over the basin and, covering your head with a towel, inhale the steam for 10 minutes. Repeat twice a day if possible. Stay in a warm room for at least 30 minutes after the inhalation to allow the mucous membranes to cool down naturally.

*See caution p. 38.

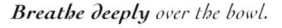

Breathe deeply *over the bowl.*

COLDS, CHILLS & FLU

Warming herbal teas soothe colds and chills as well as help relieve symptoms such as a stuffy nose, headaches, and fever. Many herbs are antibacterial and help the body to combat infection.

ELDER, YARROW & PEPPERMINT TEA

TO CLEAR A STUFFY NOSE & EASE COLD SYMPTOMS

A good basic decongestant mix to help ease congestion and clear the head.

- 10g dried elderflowers
- 10g dried yarrow*
- 5g dried peppermint

Method: Mix the herbs and make an infusion (pp. 46–7).

For the aches and pains associated with flu, add 5g each of dried boneset and dried wood betony.*

Dosage: One cup every 2–3 hours while the cold is severe; reduce to every 4 hours or 3 times a day as symptoms subside.

*See cautions pp. 9, 27.

GINGER & CINNAMON TEA

FOR COLDS & CHILLS

A warming decoction for shivery chills.

- 20g fresh ginger root, roughly chopped
- 5g powdered cinnamon

Method: Make a decoction of the ginger (pp. 48–9), adding the cinnamon midway through simmering.

Dosage: One cup every 3–4 hours.

ELECAMPANE & VERVAIN TEA

TO EASE THE SYMPTOMS OF FLU

For fever, coughing, headaches, nausea, vomiting, and aches associated with flu.

- 10g dried elecampane root*
- 5g dried licorice root*
- 5g each of dried boneset, dried yarrow,* and dried vervain,* mixed

Method: Make a decoction (pp. 48–9) using the elecampane and licorice and 750ml of water. Strain this onto the herb mixture in a teapot or lidded jug and infuse for 10 minutes.

Dosage: One cup every 3–4 hours. If depression follows the flu attack, continue taking 1 or 2 cups a day as a tonic for a couple of weeks.

*See cautions pp. 37, 37, 9, 31.

SELF-HELP SUGGESTIONS

✧

Take 5g of vitamin C daily.

Take 2 x 200mg echinacea tablets or capsules 3 times daily to combat infections.

Take 2 x 200mg garlic capsules 3 times daily if colds persist.

Eat plenty of fruit and avoid starchy foods and alcohol, which increase mucus and contribute to congestion.

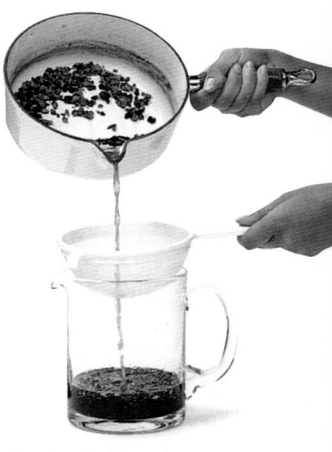

Strain the decoction *onto the dried vervain.*

CHEST PROBLEMS

Coughs can be the result of colds and flu or allergic disorders, or may simply have become a nervous habit. A persistent cough or blood-streaked phlegm will need professional treatment.

MARSH MALLOW & WILD LETTUCE TEA

FOR PERSISTENT DRY COUGHS

This tea can soothe irritant dry coughs but should not be used for productive coughs.

- 20g dried marsh mallow leaves
- 5g dried hyssop
- 5g dried wild lettuce*

Method: Mix the herbs and make an infusion (pp. 46–7).

Dosage: One cup every 4 hours, reheating each dose. *See caution p. 38.

SELF-HELP SUGGESTIONS

To relieve mild asthma attacks, take an infusion (pp. 46–7) made with 2 tbsps of dried chamomile flowers, or use 5 drops of chamomile essential oil in a steam inhalation (p. 63).

Combine 3–4 drops each of lavender and thyme essential oils with 10ml of vegetable oil. Apply 3–4 times a day as a chest rub to ease bronchial congestion.

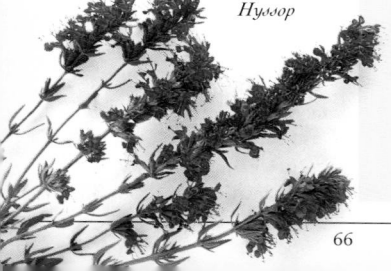

Hyssop

THYME & LICORICE SYRUP

FOR CHEST COUGHS & BRONCHITIS

Combine honey with an infusion or a decoction to make a soothing cough syrup.

- 10g licorice* juice stick
- 15g each of thyme* and hyssop, both dried
- 500g honey

Method: Gently simmer the licorice in 750ml of water until it dissolves and the mixture reduces by a third. Pour onto the herbs in a teapot, infuse for 10 minutes, then strain into a saucepan. Add the honey and simmer, stirring continuously to dissolve it. Cool and store in corked, sterilized, dark glass bottles.

Dosage: One tsp up to 6 times a day.

*See cautions pp. 37, 29.

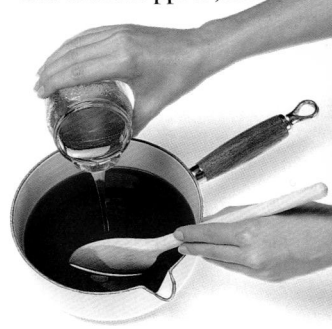

The honey dissolves to form a syrup.

ELECAMPANE & GINSENG TEA

FOR CHRONIC COUGHS

These tonic herbs help to strengthen the lungs.

- 20g dried elecampane root*
- 5g dried Korean ginseng root*
- 5g dried licorice root*

Method: Mix the herbs and make a decoction (pp. 48–9).

Dosage: One cup 3 times a day for up to 2 weeks. Reheat before each dose.

*See cautions pp. 38, 33, 37.

DIGESTIVE COMPLAINTS

Good digestion is essential for health, and its poor function can contribute to both skin and arthritic disorders. Herbal remedies make an ideal alternative to the usual battery of antacids and laxatives.

LEMON BALM & AGRIMONY TEA

FOR INDIGESTION WITH HEARTBURN, GAS, OR NAUSEA

A simple after-dinner herbal tea to calm the stomach and ease indigestion.

- 50g dried lemon balm leaves
- 25g each of agrimony and chamomile flowers, both dried
- a pinch of finely chopped fresh ginger root or powdered dried ginger, per cup

Method: Mix the herbs and make an infusion (pp. 46–7) using 2 tsps of the herbal mixture plus the ginger to 1 cup of boiling hot water.
Dosage: One cup after meals.

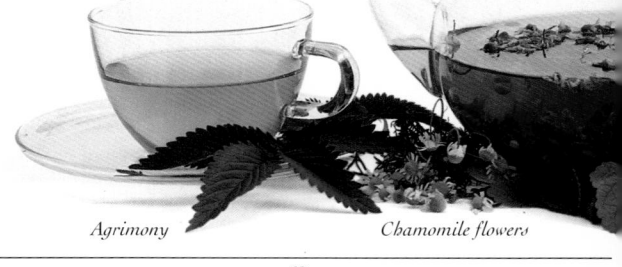

Agrimony　　　　　*Chamomile flowers*

DANDELION & LICORICE TEA

FOR CONSTIPATION

Patent herbal laxatives usually include strong purgatives, but this gentle remedy can be just as effective.

- 10g each of dandelion root and yellow dock root,* both dried
- 5g dried licorice root*
- 2g fresh ginger root, chopped

Method: Make a decoction (pp. 48–9) with all the ingredients.

Dosage: One cup before meals.

Caution: Persistent constipation can indicate more serious underlying health conditions – seek medical advice before resorting to excessive use of patent laxatives.
***See cautions pp. 39, 37.**

SELF-HELP SUGGESTIONS
⟡

Take isphaghula husks and seeds to lubricate the bowel. Soak 1 tsp in a mug of boiling water for 10–15 minutes, stir and drink first thing in the morning. Alternatively, mix the seeds with breakfast cereal and warm milk. If taking capsules, drink at least 500ml of water with each dose to prevent excessive absorption of digestive fluids.

Slippery elm and marsh mallow root soothe gastric inflammation and heartburn. Take up to 400mg as powder mixed into a paste with water, or as capsules, before meals.

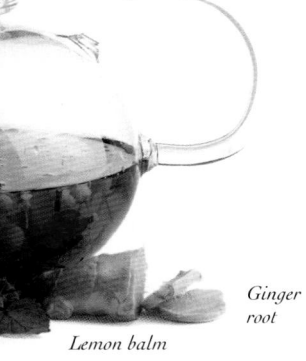

Ginger root

Lemon balm

CHAMOMILE & HOPS TEA

FOR IRRITABLE BOWEL SYNDROME

Combining sedative herbs with digestive remedies has a soothing effect on the gut.

- 30g each of chamomile flowers and meadowsweet,* both dried
- 15g each of hops* and white deadnettle, both dried
- 10g dried peppermint

Method: Mix all the herbs and make an infusion (pp. 46–7) or, for a single dose, use 2 tsps to 1 cup of boiling water.
Dosage: One cup before meals or every 3 hours if symptoms are severe.
***See cautions pp. 17, 37.**

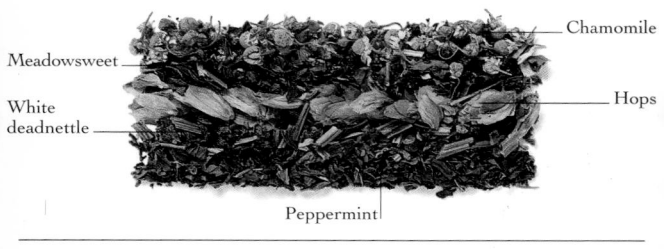

Meadowsweet

White deadnettle

Chamomile

Hops

Peppermint

MEADOWSWEET & GOTU KOLA TEA

FOR STOMACH UPSETS WITH DIARRHEA & VOMITING

To ease the symptoms of over-indulgence or food poisoning.

- 15g dried meadowsweet*
- 10g dried gotu kola
- a pinch of powdered ginger

Method: Mix all the ingredients and make an infusion (pp. 46–7).
Dosage: One cup every 2–3 hours in the acute phase.
***See caution p. 17.**

AGRIMONY & PLANTAIN TEA

FOR DIARRHEA

Orthodox diarrhea remedies often result in constipation, while herbal remedies help to calm the digestion and soothe inflamed gut membranes.

- 10g each of agrimony and common plantain, both dried
- 5g each of sage* and raspberry leaves,* both dried
- a pinch of powdered cinnamon

Method: Mix the herbs and make an infusion (pp. 46–7).
Dosage: One cup every 4 hours while symptoms persist.
Caution: Seek medical help if diarrhea persists for more than 2–3 days (more than 24 hours in babies or toddlers), or is accompanied by fever or blood and mucus in the stool.
*See cautions p. 39.

SELF-HELP SUGGESTIONS

Take 400mg–1g of powdered ginger in capsules up to 3 times a day for nausea and vomiting. Ginger candy, cookies, or ginger wine may also help.

If gastritis is linked to a hangover, take 1000mg of evening primrose oil to help normalize liver function.

For diarrhea, drink strong, cool black tea, without milk or sugar, to reduce gut inflammation.

PILEWORT

In the Middle Ages the nodular appearance of the roots led people to believe that pilewort would be a good remedy for piles. Surprisingly, the theorists were right; today this astringent herb is included in many over-the-counter remedies for hemorrhoids. Apply ointment containing the root or dried leaves to the affected area after each bowel movement and at night.

THE MOUTH & THROAT

Persistent mouth ulcers or throat infections may indicate underlying food intolerance or exhaustion. Herbs can strengthen the body's energies to combat the problem and alleviate associated irritant symptoms.

ECHINACEA & SAGE GARGLE

FOR LARYNGITIS, TONSILLITIS & SORE THROATS

These herbs have an antiseptic effect to combat infection.

- 15g dried echinacea root
- 10g each of sage* and raspberry leaves,* both dried

*See cautions p. 39.

Method: Make a decoction (pp. 48–9) with the echinacea and 750ml of water and pour it onto the herb mixture in a teapot. Infuse for 10 minutes, strain, and allow to cool.
Dosage: Gargle ½ cupful every 2–3 hours.

TEA TREE & LAVENDER OIL

FOR COLD SORES

Cold sores can develop when the immune system is under stress; antiviral herbs may help.

- 8ml tea tree oil
- 5ml lavender oil
- 12ml sweet almond oil

Method: Mix the oils in a 25ml dropper bottle. Shake well.
Application: Dab 1–2 drops onto the affected area as soon as the characteristic pricking sensation that heralds a cold sore begins. Repeat every few hours.

POT MARIGOLD MOUTHWASH

FOR MOUTH ULCERS

Mouth ulcers are often associated with digestive imbalance, candidiasis, or allergy problems. Antifungal herbs can often help.

SELF-HELP SUGGESTIONS
✧

Gargle with pure pineapple juice to ease sore throats and tonsillitis.

Make a steam inhalation (p. 63) using 2 drops each of thyme and lavender essential oils to help laryngitis and pharyngitis.

Dab a drop of clove oil directly onto a mouth ulcer; it stings, but will quickly anesthetize the associated pain.

For recurrent cold sores or mouth ulcers, take 1g of vitamin C per day and 200mg of garlic 3 times daily. Take 200mg of echinacea 3 times daily to combat infection.

• 15g each of dried pot marigold petals and fresh or dried rosemary

Method: Make an infusion (pp. 46–7). Allow it to cool thoroughly, then strain.
Dosage: Use as a mouthwash every 2–3 hours during the acute phase. Repeat 2–3 times a day for less severe mouth inflammations.

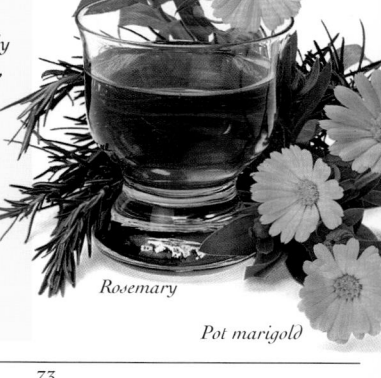

Rosemary

Pot marigold

EYE & EAR PROBLEMS

In the past herbs were often taken to improve both sight and hearing; today their use is more generally limited to combating simple eye and ear inflammations and other minor disorders.

POT MARIGOLD & RASPBERRY EYEBATH

FOR CONJUNCTIVITIS & SORE EYES

Soothing, astringent herbs can cool the burning eye sensation associated with hay fever, conjunctivitis, and allergies.

- 10g each of pot marigold petals and elderflowers, both dried
- 5g dried raspberry leaves

Keep the head
tilted back.

Method: Mix the herbs and simmer in 500ml of water for 5–10 minutes to sterilize the mixture. Strain and allow to cool thoroughly.

Application: Pour a little into a sterile eyebath and bathe the eye thoroughly. If both eyes are infected, sterilize the eyebath and use a fresh dose of infusion for the other eye. Repeat every 1–2 hours in acute cases.

Caution: Eye infections can be very contagious – do not share face towels or cloths within the household.

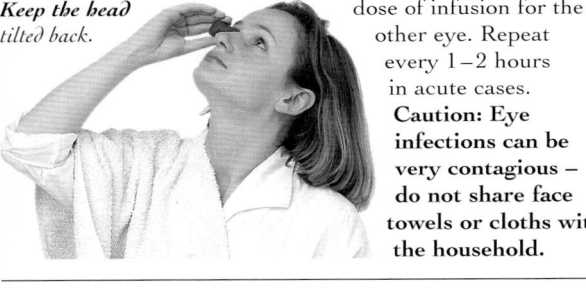

ST. JOHN'S WORT EARDROPS
FOR EARACHE

Herbal eardrops can help to ease the pain of earache, which is often associated with upper respiratory tract infections.

- 15ml St. John's wort oil
- 10ml sweet almond oil

Method: Mix the oils in a 25ml sterilized, dark glass dropper bottle. Shake well.
Application: Put 2 drops into the ear and cover with a cotton plug. Repeat 3 times a day.

Caution: Never put anything in the ear if the drum is perforated. Seek medical help if symptoms persist for more than 24 hours.

SELF-HELP SUGGESTIONS
❖

Apply pot marigold cream to sties 2–3 times daily, and take echinacea and garlic to combat infections (p. 65).

Apply used fennel, elderflower, or chamomile teabags to tired eyes.

Mix 2ml each of lavender and tea tree essential oils in 20ml of sweet almond oil. Massage around the ear and back of the neck to relieve ear infections.

Dark circles under the eyes can indicate food allergies. Look at your diet and drink agrimony tea (p. 68) to aid digestion.

Hold used, warm chamomile or St. John's wort teabags to the ear to relieve painful earache.

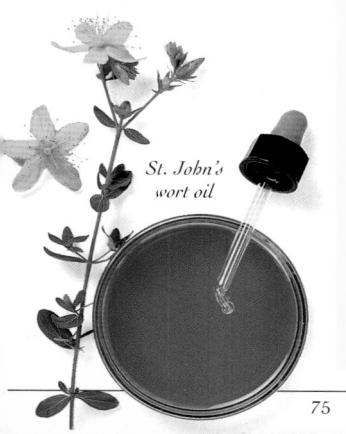

St. John's
wort oil

HEAD & NERVE PAINS

Headaches can suggest problems elsewhere in the body,
so finding the cause is vital. Pain behind the eyes can
be due to sluggish digestion (pp. 68–71), while pain
between the eyes may indicate sinus problems (p. 65).

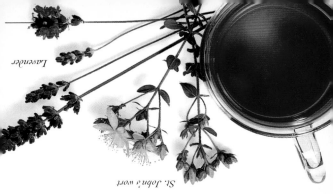

Lavender

St. John's wort

ST. JOHN'S WORT & LAVENDER TEA

FOR NEURALGIA

Neuralgia often affects the
facial nerves. Used in addition
to topical treatments, herbal
tea can offer soothing relief.

- 15g dried St. John's wort *
- 10g dried lavender flowers

Method: Mix the herbs and
make an infusion (pp. 46–7).
Dosage: Sip a large mugful
every 2–3 hours while
symptoms are severe.
❈ See caution p. 19.

WOOD BETONY & CHAMOMILE TEA
FOR TENSION HEADACHES

Taking time to make calming teas can also help counter tension and stress.

- 60g dried wood betony*
- 30g dried chamomile flowers
- 10g dried lavender flowers

SELF-HELP SUGGESTIONS

To help ease a tension headache, soak in a relaxing herbal bath with 4 drops of lavender or chamomile essential oil added.

Mix 20 drops of lavender essential oil in 10ml sweet almond oil and massage into the nape of neck and temples at the first signs of a migraine.

For neuralgia, apply fresh lemon juice or slices of lemon to the affected area. A hot compress soaked in an infusion (pp. 46–7) made from equal amounts of St. John's wort and vervain may also help.

Method: Mix the herbs and use 2 tsps to 1 cup of boiling water to make an infusion (pp. 46–7). **Dosage:** One cup every hour while the headache continues. **Caution: Persistent headaches can be a symptom of high blood pressure or more serious conditions. Seek medical advice if headaches are recurrent or sustained.** *See caution p. 27.

FEVERFEW

This herb is known to be anti-inflammatory, analgesic, antispasmodic, and effective for easing migraines and arthritis. Eating a few fresh leaves a day can help prevent migraine attacks, but may cause mouth ulcers. Take 200mg up to 3 times daily. Not to be taken by those on blood-thinning drugs and is best avoided in pregnancy.

SKIN PROBLEMS

Herbalists generally prefer to treat skin problems with cleansing remedies taken internally rather than relying exclusively on external creams or lotions, which may only superficially clear the problem.

BURDOCK & HEARTSEASE TEA

FOR IRRITANT SKIN CONDITIONS

By cleansing the body of toxins, this infusion may help skin disorders such as eczema and psoriasis.

- 10g each of burdock root and yellow dock* root, dried
- 10g dried heartsease
- 5g dried skullcap

Method: Make a decoction with the burdock and yellow dock (pp. 48–9). Strain onto the dried herbs in a teapot or jug and infuse for 10 minutes.
Dosage: ½ cupful, 3 times a day before meals.
***See caution p. 39.**

AGRIMONY & MEADOWSWEET TEA

FOR HIVES & SKIN RASHES RELATED TO FOOD ALLERGIES

Herbs can help the digestion and thus any skin irritation if the problem is food-related.

- 15g dried agrimony
- 10g dried meadowsweet*
- 5g dried wood betony*

Method: Mix the herbs and make an infusion (pp. 46–7).
Dosage: One cupful, 3 times a day before meals.
***See cautions pp. 17, 27.**

LAVENDER & YARROW FACIAL

FOR ACNE

Steaming the face deep-cleanses inflamed pores and pimples common in acne.

- 10g dried lavender flowers
- 10g dried yarrow (flowers, if available, or leaves)
- 10g dried elderflowers

Method: Mix the herbs in a basin. Pour over boiling water as for an inhalation (p. 63).

Application: Allow the steam to engulf the face for 5 – 10 minutes. Repeat once a day.

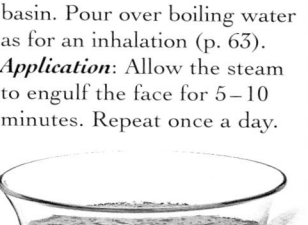

Yarrow   Lavender

SELF-HELP SUGGESTIONS
◇

Make a cleansing lotion for acne with 25ml each of distilled witch hazel and rosewater and 5 drops of tea tree essential oil. Apply twice daily with cotton.

Use chickweed cream on eczema and pot marigold cream on dry skin.

Treat fungal skin infections, such as athlete's foot or ringworm, with tea tree or pot marigold creams.

For psoriasis of the scalp, make an infusion of rosemary (pp. 46–7) and rinse through the hair after shampooing.

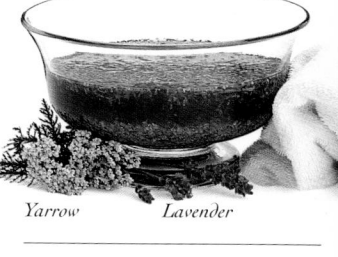

EVENING PRIMROSE
Oil from the seeds of this plant is rich in gamma-linolenic acid, an essential fatty acid vital for many bodily functions. Its lack can contribute to such problems as chronic skin conditions, arthritis, and menstrual irregularities. Take 500–1000mg daily for at least 3 months.

WOMEN'S HEALTH

Menstrual pain or those "difficult days" caused by premenstrual tension affect many women, who often find little relief in orthodox medicine. Herbs have a long tradition of easing menstrual irregularities.

MARSH MALLOW & YARROW TEA

FOR BLADDER & URINARY TRACT INFLAMMATION

Cystitis often follows intercourse if bacteria enter the urinary tract accidentally.

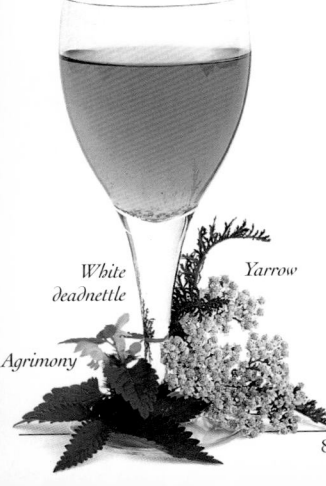

White deadnettle

Yarrow

Agrimony

• 10g dried marsh mallow root
• 5g each of agrimony, white deadnettle, celery seed,* and yarrow*, all dried

Method: Soak the marsh mallow in 500ml of water overnight. Heat the mixture to boiling point and pour onto the dried herbs in a teapot or jug. Infuse for 10 minutes, then strain.

Dosage: One cupful, 3 times a day before meals.

Caution: Seek medical help if symptoms do not ease within a few days or if there is any risk of kidney involvement (characterized by fever and midback pain).
*See cautions pp. 36, 9.

St. John's Wort & Raspberry Tea

For menstrual pain

A soothing combination of herbs to ease menstrual pain.

St. John's wort

Peppermint

Raspberry leaf

- 15g each of St. John's wort* and raspberry leaves,* dried
- 5g dried peppermint

Method: Mix the herbs and make an infusion (pp. 46–7).

Dosage: One cup every 2–3 hours, up to 6 times a day, while symptoms persist. For heavy periods, replace the peppermint with 10g of dried yarrow* or white deadnettle.
See cautions pp. 19, 39, 9.

Self-help Suggestions

Take 500–1000mg of evening primrose oil (p. 79) daily for menstrual problems.

Take up to 600mg of dang gui (p. 32) in capsule form 3 times daily for premenstrual problems, an irregular cycle, or for menopausal symptoms.

Use tea tree or pot marigold cream or suppositories for yeast infections.

Always drink plenty of water and avoid alcohol during attacks of cystitis.

Chaste Tree

This herb, also known as Agnus castus, acts on the pituitary gland, which regulates the production of female sex hormones. The berries were traditionally regarded as a female aphrodisiac, but believed to have the opposite effect on men. To ease premenstrual tension, take 10 drops of tincture each morning, increasing to 20 drops for the 10 days before a period.

GROWING OLDER

Aging brings its own health problems, from difficult menopausal years and prostate disorders to the mental confusion often associated with extreme old age. In many cases, suitable herbs can help.

SAGE & VERVAIN TEA
FOR RELIEF FROM MENOPAUSAL PROBLEMS

An herbal mixture to ease hot flashes, night sweats, and emotional upsets associated with menopause.

- 25g each of vervain,* sage,* and raspberry leaves,* all dried
- 10g each of lavender flowers and St. John's wort,* both dried

Method: Mix the herbs and use 2 tsps to 1 cup of

boiling water to make an infusion (pp. 46–7).
Dosage: One cup up to 4 times a day.
**See cautions pp. 31, 39, 39, 19.*

St. John's wort

Lavender

DEADNETTLE & GINSENG TEA

FOR PROSTATE GLAND PROBLEMS

Prostate gland inflammation and enlargement are common disorders in older men.

- 10g each of Siberian ginseng and echinacea root, both dried
- 15g dried white deadnettle

Method: Make a decoction (pp. 48–9) with the ginseng and echinacea and 750ml of water. Strain onto the white deadnettle in a teapot or jug and infuse for 10 minutes.

Dosage: One cup 3 times daily before meals.

Caution: Because of the risk of prostate cancer, thorough medical examination is always recommended. Do not stop taking orthodox medication for prostate problems without consulting your doctor.

SELF-HELP SUGGESTIONS

Apply pot marigold or vitamin E creams directly to the vagina to ease menopausal dryness. Regular intercourse helps to maintain a healthy vaginal lining.

Eat a handful of pumpkin seeds daily; they are rich in zinc, which is essential for the male hormonal system.

Drink a ginger decoction (pp. 48–9) or a yarrow infusion (pp. 46–7) for poor circulation.

GINKGO

This plant significantly improves cerebral as well as peripheral circulation and has been successfully used in Germany to speed recovery following brain surgery. It is widely promoted as an antiaging remedy since it prevents the arteries in the brain from hardening, a common cause of confusion in the elderly. Take 5ml of tincture 3 times daily.

PREGNANCY & BIRTH

The modern approach to childbirth gives women little opportunity to benefit from the many herbs traditionally used to ease labor and aid a swift delivery, but herbs can help in pregnancy and after the birth.

Note: Many herbs should be avoided in pregnancy as they can stimulate the uterus or cause fetal abnormalities. Of the herbs mentioned in this book, do not use the following at all: chamomile essential oil (pp. 22–3), devil's claw (*Harpagophytum procumbens*), feverfew (*Tanacetum parthenium*). Do not take large or therapeutic doses of the following: celery seed (*Apium graveolens*), Chinese Angelica (*Angelica polymorpha*), cinnamon (*Cinnamomum zeylanicum*), elder bark (*Sambucus nigra*), fennel (*Foeniculum officinalis*), ginseng (*Panax ginseng*), lavender (*Lavandula angustifolia*), licorice (*Glycyrrhiza glabra*), nutmeg (*Myristica fragrans*), sage (*Salvia officinalis*), thyme (*Thymus vulgaris*), vervain (*Verbena officinalis*), wood betony (*Stachys officinalis*), and yarrow (*Achillea millefolium*). Consult a practitioner before using medication or any other herbs.

GINGER & CHAMOMILE TEA

FOR MORNING SICKNESS

Morning sickness affects many women in early pregnancy.

- 15g fresh ginger root
- 10g dried chamomile flowers
- 5g each lemon balm and peppermint, both dried

Method: Make a decoction (pp. 48–9) with the ginger and 750ml of water. Simmer for 15 minutes, then pour onto the dried herbs in a teapot or jug and infuse for 10 minutes. Strain into a warmed vacuum flask or jug.

Dosage: Keep the flask by the bed and drink a cup on waking, before getting out of bed.

CHILDBIRTH KIT

Herbal teas containing wood betony, chamomile, or raspberry leaf with a few cloves or ground nutmeg can be helpful in labor, but may not be welcome in all maternity wards. If they are, keep a mug of hot tea close at hand and sip as required. Skullcap tea can soothe if the mother is anxious. Tablets, oils, and creams are often more acceptable. A herbal birth kit should contain:

• **1ml of clove oil diluted in 10ml of vegetable oil**: Massage into the lower abdomen during labor to help encourage contractions.
• **1ml of lavender oil diluted in 10ml of vegetable oil**: Firmly massage into the lower back during the harder stages of labor.
• **Homeopathic Arnica 6x**: Dissolve 1 tablet on the tongue every 15–30 minutes immediately after delivery to speed recovery.
• **Infused oils of St. John's wort and comfrey**: Add 20ml of each to postpartum baths to soothe any bruising or tearing of the perineum.
• **Comfrey or witch hazel cream**: Apply to the perineum

to speed healing and soothe.
• **Pot marigold cream**: Inexpert sucking by small babies can lead to sore nipples. Use the cream to relieve discomfort, but wipe nipples before feeding the baby.

SELF-HELP SUGGESTIONS

❖

To ease mastitis, insert a clean, slightly crushed cabbage leaf between breast and bra.

Chinese angelica root (dang gui, p. 32) is traditionally used as a tonic after childbirth. Take ½ tsp (2.5ml) of tincture in water 3 times a day or add small pieces to stews and casseroles (but remove it before serving).

BABIES & CHILDREN

*Gentle herbal remedies can be ideal for children —
turn the remedy into a game by giving it in drop doses
on the tongue using a pipette. Add a little honey or
peppermint* if desired, to counter the bitter taste.*

Note: Seek immediate medical help for severe diarrhea or vomiting, a
fever of 102°F (39°C) or above, convulsions, breathing difficulties, unusual
drowsiness, or high-pitched crying. Do not give babies under
6 months any medicine internally without professional advice.
Dosage: All doses on pp. 86–9 are suitable for babies and children.
If using remedies elsewhere in the book for children, reduce the dose as
follows: for toddlers under 2 years, use a fifth of the adult dose, increasing
gradually to a quarter of the adult dose at 3 or 4 (depending on the size
of the child); use a third of the adult dose at 6 or 7, and a half at
8 or 9, increasing to the full adult dose at puberty.
*Children under 1 should not be given honey or peppermint.

CHAMOMILE TEA & BATH

FOR SLEEPLESSNESS

*Drinking this infusion and
adding it to a bath can help
to encourage sleep.*

- 15g dried chamomile flowers
- 5g dried lemon balm

Method: Mix the herbs and
make an infusion (pp. 46–7).
Application: For bottle-fed

babies, add 3 tsps of the tea
to the nighttime feeding and
strain 200ml of the infusion
into the child's bath water at
night. Children age 2 and
over should drink 50–100ml
of the tea at bedtime. Store
any remaining infusion in the
refrigerator, reheat, and use
the following night.

CHAMOMILE & SAGE GUM RUB

FOR TEETHING PAINS

Ease the teething pains common in babies of 4 months or younger with this soothing rub.

- 4 drops chamomile oil
- 2 drops sage oil
- 2 drops rosemary oil
- 20ml sunflower or almond oil

Method: Add the essential oils to the sunflower or almond oil in a 20ml sterilized, dark glass bottle and shake well.

Application: Smear a small amount of the oil on your finger and very gently rub the baby's gums with it. Repeat the procedure 3 or 4 times a day. An infused oil of garden mint (pp. 50–1) makes a good base instead of sunflower or almond oil.

SELF-HELP SUGGESTIONS
✧

For cradle cap, bathe the affected area in an infusion of heartsease (pp. 46–7).

To soothe diaper rash, after each diaper change apply 5 drops tea tree essential oil mixed with 10ml infused comfrey oil.

For nits and head lice, comb a few drops of tea tree essential oil through the hair or add 10 drops to 500ml of warm water and rinse through after shampooing.

DILL

Generations of parents have relied on dill to ease their baby's gas and colic. A weak infusion of dill seeds helps provide relief for baby (and parents!). Dill increases milk production for nursing mothers. It can also be added to cough and cold remedies. Avoid the use of alcohol in any preparations intended for small children and infants.

CATNIP & ELDERFLOWER TEA

FOR FEVERS

Childhood fevers can be sudden and dramatic but will usually subside within a few hours.

- 30g dried catnip
- 10g dried elderflowers
- 10g dried yarrow*

Method: Mix the herbs, measure out 10g, and make an infusion (pp. 46–7) using 500ml of boiling water.
Dosage: Half a cup every 2 hours to children aged 2 and under, increasing to 1 cup 3 times a day for 6 year olds and over. Sweeten with a little honey if required but do not give honey to children under 1. Keep the child cool by removing clothing and sponging with lukewarm water. Encourage the child to drink plenty of fresh fruit juices to increase intake of vitamin C.
Caution: Seek medical help if symptoms persist or the fever rises above 102°F (39°C).
*See caution p. 9.

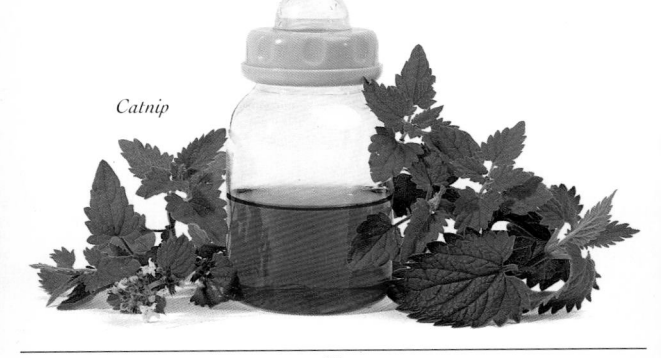

Catnip

AGRIMONY & CATNIP TEA

FOR NAUSEA, COLIC, DIARRHEA & STOMACH UPSETS

Agrimony and catnip can bring soothing relief for childhood tummy upsets and related problems.

- 10g each of agrimony and catnip, both dried
- 5g each of meadowsweet* and dill seeds, both dried

Method: Mix the herbs and make an infusion (pp. 46–47).
Dosage: A quarter to 1 cup 3 times a day (see note on dosage p. 86). For upset stomach with nausea and vomiting, replace the agrimony with 10g of dried wood betony.
*See caution p. 17.

SELF-HELP SUGGESTIONS
❖

For coughs and nasal congestion, mix 2 drops of thyme or hyssop essential oil into 1 tsp of vegetable oil. Rub a small amount on the chest or pour into a saucer of water at the bedside so that the child can inhale the fumes.

Give 80–400g echinacea, 2 times daily for childhood colds and infections. Tablets can be crushed for smaller children.

To ease constipation, give a glass of sweetened prune juice morning and evening.

CATNIP

Well-known to gardeners as a favorite herb with cats, who will roll ecstatically in the plant, catnip is ideal to grow if you have small children in the house. The herb soothes digestion, helps to reduce body temperature in fever, and can relieve nasal congestion. Although related to peppermint, it has none of that herb's irritant qualities and is perfectly safe in teas for childhood tummy upsets, fevers, congestion (including middle ear problems), and diarrhea.

HERBAL MEDICINE CHEST

Herbs make an ideal alternative to the patent synthetic drugs that we usually reach for to treat minor ailments or accidents.

THE BASIC FIRST-AID KIT

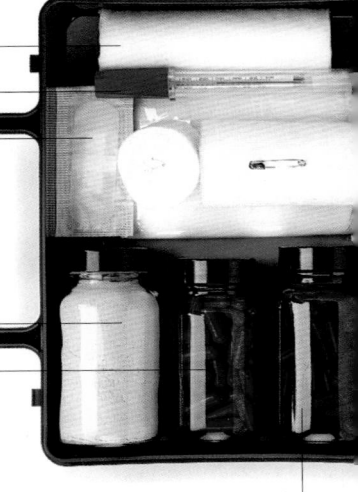

Bandage

Thermometer

Adhesive bandages

Slippery elm powder *soothes stomach inflammation. It can also be taken for irritant coughs. Mix 1 tsp with a little water to make a paste, and take up to 3 times a day before meals.*

Garlic tablets *ease congestion and coughs, boost the immune system, and help reduce cholesterol level. Take the equivalent of 2000mg daily. Low doses taken regularly can help improve digestive function in the elderly (p. 32).*

Echinacea tablets *combat colds, flu, and other infections (p. 32). Take 2 x 200mg 3 times a day.*

Chickweed cream can be applied to eczema, minor burns, sunburn, and insect stings. Use overnight for drawing out splinters and on boils.

Arnica cream improves circulation and encourages healing. Use on chilblains, bruises, and sprains (but not on broken skin).

Comfrey cream speeds up tissue growth and repair. Apply liberally to bruises, sprains, fractures, and small cracked bones. (Do not use on broken skin.)

Clove essential oil soothes insect stings and toothache. Apply to the gum with a cotton swab.

Thyme syrup for chest infections and coughs (p. 28). Take 5ml 3 times a day.

Passion flower tablets make a helpful sedative. For anxiety, take 2 x 200mg up to 3 times a day. For insomnia (p. 56), take 3 x 200mg 30 minutes before bedtime.

Distilled witch hazel is highly astringent, anti-inflammatory, and it stops bleeding. Use as a cooling lotion for cuts and scrapes, minor burns, sunburn, bruises, insect stings, varicose veins, and piles.

Lavender essential oil in a vegetable oil base makes a good rub for muscle pains and headaches. Use on bites, minor burns, and sunburn (p. 20).

Tea tree essential oil is antiseptic and antifungal. Apply pure oil to cuts or fungal skin infections. Use 3–4 drops on a tampon for up to 3 hours to combat yeast infections.

Evening primrose oil capsules are a good hangover cure, helping to restore liver function. Take 2–3g the morning after (p. 74). Use the oil on skin rashes.

TRAVEL KIT

A roll-up bag will hold first-aid essentials and is easily portable. For dosages, see chart opposite.

Crystallized ginger for motion sickness.

Chamomile teabags, soothing for tired eyes.

Arnica or comfrey cream for bruises and strains.

Arnica 6X helps counter shock.

St. John's wort oil eases burns.

Lavender essential oil, useful for heat stroke and sunburn.

Siberian ginseng capsules to counter jet lag.

Meadowsweet tincture for stomach upsets (p. 16).

St. John's wort and pot marigold tincture treats cuts and grazes.

Agrimony and gotu kola tincture, a diarrhea remedy.

AILMENT	REMEDY
BRUISES	Cool with ice cubes of distilled witch hazel or apply arnica or comfrey creams, infused oils, or ointments.
MINOR BURNS, SUNBURN, AND SCALDS	Cool minor burns under running cold water or with ice cubes of witch hazel. Apply 1ml of lavender essential oil diluted in a glass of cold water, or pure St. John's wort oil. Seek medical advice for serious or deep burns (more than 1cm in diameter).
MINOR CUTS AND SCRAPES	Apply tea tree, pot marigold, or St. John's wort creams, or a compress soaked in 10ml of St. John's wort and pot marigold tincture in 250ml of hot water.
DIARRHEA	Take 2 tsp (10ml) of agrimony and gotu kola tincture in a glass of warm water every 2–3 hours.
HEAT STROKE	Mix 1 tsp each of salt and sugar in a tumbler of water and drink. Bathe the forehead with 1ml of lavender essential oil diluted in a glass of cold water.
INSECT BITES AND STINGS	Remove any sting with tweezers and gently press the poison from the wound. Apply slices of raw onion, freshly crushed common plantain leaves, or 1ml of lavender essential oil diluted in a glass of water.
JET LAG	Take 2 x 200mg capsules of Siberian ginseng for 3 days before traveling and 2 days afterward. Drink chamomile tea in-flight and save the used teabags as eye pads to relieve the irritation caused by the dry atmosphere.
NOSEBLEEDS	Use a distilled witch hazel compress on the nose. Insert a cotton swab moistened with yarrow tincture.
SHOCK	Take 1 tablet of homeopathic arnica 6X every 30 minutes.
SPLINTERS	Extract the splinter with a sterile needle and apply tea tree or pot marigold cream. Use chickweed or slippery elm ointment to draw out stubborn splinters.
SPRAINS AND STRAINS	Apply a cabbage leaf, arnica, or comfrey cream, or apply a cloth soaked in hot rosemary infusion as a compress.
MOTION SICKNESS	Take 2 x 200mg capsules of ginger or chew crystallized ginger 30 minutes before starting the trip.

INDEX

Main entries in **bold**.

A·B

acne 79
agrimony **10–11**, 43, 75
 first aid 92, 93
 key remedies 68, 71, 78,
  80, 89
allergies (food) 10, 78
anxiety 18, 60
arnica 55, 85, 91, 92, 93
arthritis 59, 79
asthma 66
athlete's foot 14, 79
bladder inflammation 80
boneset **37**, 43, 64, 65
bronchitis 67
bruises 93
burdock **36**, 43, 59, 78
burns and scalds 93

C

cabbage **34**, 49, 85, 93
capsules 52
catnip (*Nepeta cataria*)
 42, 43, 88, **89**
celery **36**, 42, 43, 59, 80, 84
chamomile **22–3**, 42, 43,
 54, 55, 75
 first aid 92, 93
 key remedies 66, 68, 70,
  77, 84, 85, 86, 87
chaste tree (*Vitex agnus
 castus*) 43, **81**
chickweed (*Stellaria media*)
 42, 43, 51, 55, 79, 91, 93
Chinese angelica *see đang gui*
cinnamon **35**, 64, 71, 84
circulation 8, 26, 83
clove (*Syzygium
 aromaticum*) 73, 85, 91
cold sores 72

colds and chills 64
colic 87, 89
comfrey (*Symphytum
 officinale*) 43, 51, 55, 85, 87
 first aid 91, 92, 93
congestion 10, 62–3
conjunctivitis 16, 74
constipation 69
coughs 66–7
cradle cap 87
creams 55
cuts and scrapes 93
cystitis 80, 81

D·E·F

damiana **33**, 61
dandelion **40**, 42, 43, 54,
 62, 69
dandruff 24
đang gui **32**, 81, 85
decoctions 48–9
depression 18
devil's claw
 (*Harpagophytum
 procumbens*) 52, **59**, 84
diaper rash 87
diarrhea 28, 70, 71, 89, 93
dill (*Anethum graveolens*)
 42, 43, 44, **87**, 89
earache 75
echinacea **36**, 43, 52, 54,
 65, 73, 75, 89, 90
 key remedies 72, 83
eczema 10, 14, 78, 79
elder **39**, 43, 53, 55, 63, 75, 84
 key remedies 59, 62, 64,
  74, 79, 88
elecampane **37**, 42, 43, 54,
 65, 67
essential oils 54
eucalyptus **37**
evening primrose (*Oenothera
 biennis*) 43, 55, 71, **79**, 81, 91
eyes, sore 74

fatigue 28, 61
fennel **35**, 42, 43, 53, 75, 84
feverfew (*Tanacetum
 parthenium*) 42, 43, **77**, 84
fevers 88, 89
flu 64, 65

G·H·I·J

garlic **36**, 43, 45, 52, 52,
 65, 73, 75, 90
ginger **40**, 71, 83
 first aid 92, 93
 key remedies 64, 68, 69,
  70, 84
ginkgo (*Ginkgo biloba*) 43,
 52, **83**
gotu kola **32**, 61, 70, 92, 93
hay fever 8, 22, 62, 74
headaches 76, 77
head lice 87
heartburn 69
heartsease **40**, 43, 55, 78, 87
heat stroke 93
hops **37**, 43, 70
hyssop **37**, 42, 43, 54, 89
 key remedies 62, 66, 67
Indian pennywort *see
 gotu kola*
indigestion 68, 69
infused oils 50–1
infusions 46–7, 49
insect stings 30, 93
insomnia 20, 60, 61
ipecac (*Cephaelis
 ipecacuanha*) 54
irritable bowel
 syndrome 28, 70
isphaghula **39**, 69
jet lag 93
juices 54

K·L·M·N

Korean ginseng **33**, 52,
 67, 84

GLOSSARY

Bitter – digestive stimulant.
Carminative – relieves flatulence, digestive colic, and gastric discomfort.
Demulcent – soothes and softens damaged or inflamed surfaces, such as the gastric mucous membranes.

Febrifuge – reduces fever.
Nervine – affects the nervous system.
Saponin – a soaplike plant constituent.
Styptic – stops external bleeding.
Tonic – restores and nourishes the body.

USEFUL ADDRESSES

ASSOCIATIONS & PROFESSIONAL BODIES:

American Herb Association, P.O. Box 1673, Nevada City, CA 95959

Herb Research Foundation, 1007 Pearl St., Ste. 200, Boulder, CO 80302

American Herbalists Guild, Box 1683, Soquel, CA 95073

Canadian Association of Herbal Practitioners, 921 17th Avenue SW, Calgary, Alta. T2T 0A4

Ontario Herbalists Association, 11 Winthrop Pl., Stoney Creek, Ont. L8G 3M3

MAIL ORDER HERB SUPPLIERS:

East Coast Herbs, 118 16th Street, South, Ste. 200, Nashville, TN 37 203
The Body Shop by Mail, 45 Horsehill Rd., Cedar Knolls, NJ 07927
Gaia Herbs, 62 Old Littleton Rd., Harvard, MA 01451
Gaia Garden Herbal Apothecary, 2672 W. Broadway, Vancouver, BC V6K 2G3
Herbs Etc., 1340 Rufina Circle, Santa Fe, NM 87501
International Herbs Co., 31 St. Andrews, Toronto, Ont. M5T 1K7
Catnip Acres Herb Nursery, 67 Christian Street, Oxford, CT 06483-1224
Companion Plants, 7247 N. Coolville Ridge Road, Athens, OH 45701
Earthstar Herb Gardens, P.O. Box 1022, Chino Valley, AZ86323

ACKNOWLEDGMENTS

Dorling Kindersley would like to thank Fiona Cromley and Susan Minter at the Chelsea Physic Garden; Neal's Yard; Penny Warren, Rosie Pearson, Nell, and Monica for editorial assistance; Sarah Ereira for compiling the index; Geraldine Cooney for proofreading; Michael Wise, Irene Pavitt, and, as always, Phoebe Todd-Naylor.
PICTURE CREDITS
Main photography by Steve Gorton. Additional photography by Sandra Lousada (p. 58), Andy Crawford, Dave King, Neil Fletcher, Matthew Ward, Martin Cameron, and Peter Anderson. Line art illustrations by Gilly Newman.